T0211761

Palgrave Global Media Policy and Business

Series Editors: **Professor Petros Iosifidis, Professor Jeanette Steemers** and **Professor Gerald Sussman**

Editorial Board: **Sandra Braman, Peter Dahlgren, Terry Flew, Charles Fombad, Manuel Alejandro Guerrero, Alison Harcourt, Robin Mansell, Richard Maxwell, Toby Miller, Zizi Papacharissi, Stylianos Papathanassopoulos, Caroline Pauwels, Robert Picard, Kiran Prasad, Marc Raboy, Chang Yong Son, Miklos Suksod, Kenton T. Wilkinson, Sugmin Youn**

This innovative series examines the wider social, political, economic and technological changes arising from the globalization of the media and communications industries and assesses their impact on matters of business practice, regulation and policy. Considering media convergence, industry concentration, and new communications practices, the series makes reference to the paradigmatic shift from a system based on national decision-making and the traditions of public service in broadcast and telecommunications delivery to one that is demarcated by commercialization, privatization and monopolization. Bearing in mind this shift, and based on a multi-disciplinary approach, the series tackles three key questions: To what extent do new media developments require changes in regulatory philosophy and objectives? To what extent do new technologies and changing media consumption require changes in business practices and models? And to what extent does privatization alter the creative freedom and public accountability of media enterprises?

Steven Barnett & Judith Townend (*editors*)
MEDIA POWER AND PLURALITY
From Hyperlocal to High-Level Policy

Abu Bhuiyan
INTERNET GOVERNANCE AND THE GLOBAL SOUTH
Demand for a New Framework

Benedetta Brevini
PUBLIC SERVICE BROADCASTING ONLINE
A Comparative European Policy Study of PSB 2.0

Karen Donders, Caroline Pauwels and Jan Loisen (*editors*)
PRIVATE TELEVISION IN WESTERN EUROPE
Content, Markets, Policies

Tim Dwyer
CONVERGENT MEDIA AND PRIVACY

Tom Evens, Petros Iosifidis and Paul Smith
THE POLITICAL ECONOMY OF TELEVISION SPORTS RIGHTS

Terry Flew, Petros Iosifidis and Jeanette Steemers
GLOBAL MEDIA AND NATIONAL POLICIES
The Return of the State

Manuel Guerrero and Mireya Márquez-Ramírez (*editors*)
MEDIA SYSTEMS AND COMMUNICATION POLICIES IN LATIN AMERICA

Petros Iosifidis
GLOBAL MEDIA AND COMMUNICATION POLICY
An International Perspective

John Lent and Michelle Amazeen (*editors*)
KEY THINKERS IN CRITICAL COMMUNICATION SCHOLARSHIP
From the Pioneers to the Next Generation

Michael Starks
THE DIGITAL TELEVISION REVOLUTION
Origins to Outcomes

Peggy Valcke, Miklos Sükösd and Robert Picard (*editors*)
MEDIA PLURALISM AND DIVERSITY
Concepts, Risks and Global Trends

Tim Dwyer
CONVERGENT MEDIA AND PRIVACY

Terry Flew, Petros Iosifidis and Jeanette Steemers (*editors*)
GLOBAL MEDIA AND NATIONAL POLICIES
The Return of the State

Mike Milne
THE TRANSFORMATION OF TELEVISION SPORT
New Methods, New Rules

Palgrave Global Media Policy and Business
Series Standing Order ISBN 978–1–137–27329–1 (hardback)
978–1–137–36718–1 (paperback)
(*outside North America only*)

You can receive future titles in this series as they are published by placing a standing order. Please contact your bookseller or, in case of difficulty, write to us at the address below with your name and address, the title of the series and the ISBN quoted above.

Customer Services Department, Macmillan Distribution Ltd, Houndmills, Basingstoke, Hampshire RG21 6XS, England

---

The Transformation of Television Sport

New Methods, New Rules

Mike Milne
Media Executive, UK

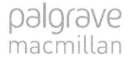

First published 2016 by
PALGRAVE MACMILLAN

Palgrave Macmillan in the UK is an imprint of Macmillan Publishers Limited, registered in England, company number 785998, of Houndmills, Basingstoke, Hampshire, RG21 6XS.

Palgrave Macmillan in the US is a division of Nature America, Inc., One New York Plaza, Suite 4500, New York, NY 10004-1562.

Palgrave Macmillan is the global academic imprint of the above companies and has companies and representatives throughout the world.

ISBN 978–1–349–71904–4
E-PDF ISBN: 978–1–137–55911–1
DOI: 10.1057/9781137559111

Distribution in the UK, Europe and the rest of the world is by Palgrave Macmillan®, a division of Macmillan Publishers Limited, registered in England, company number 785998, of Houndmills, Basingstoke, Hampshire RG21 6XS.

A catalog record for this book is available from the Library of Congress.

A catalogue record for the book is available from the British Library.

To Annette and Zoë, my anchor and inspiration, who kindly tolerate my grumpiness when Chelsea lose

Contents

Figures and Tables

Figures

Tables

Foreword

Over the last couple of decades, one of the most significant trends in the global audiovisual market has been the growth of sports coverage. This has gone hand in hand with the general commercialisation of sport and has developed at an ever increasing pace since the worldwide liberalisation of audiovisual markets. Hence, the growing number of works – though still limited – that emphasise the triadic relationship between sports, the media and corporate interests. Mike Milne's comprehensive book examines fundamental changes to the television sport supply chain by tackling increasingly influential upstream activities – technology, broadcasting rights and regulation – together with the downstream impact of transformations on broadcasters, media providers, independent sports, independent production companies and the day-to-day work of producers and directors, the final intermediaries. The role of technology in increasing the volume and scope of sports content that can be produced and distributed is reviewed but the author is careful to avoid technological determinism.

The volume also takes a historical perspective. Alongside considering the incursion of marketing and promotional strategies it addresses a gap in the political economy coverage of television sport by comparing the various technological, economic and political developments in the US and UK since WWII. It also considers copyright and intellectual property; it focuses on the role of regulation from national and international level broadcasting policies such as the list of protected events; it deals with a range of challenges now faced by broadcasters and media providers including the growing competition for the acquisition of broadcasting rights, and identifies crucial trends in independent sports production. In effect, this competent book is interested in three fundamental questions: who produces television sport; why it is produced the way it is; and what the consequences might be. It provides a useful case study from the English Premier League and the escalation in the value of football rights, but also draws valuable examples from the American National Football League as well as Formula 1.

The television sport sector has been transformed beyond recognition. It has become a big, global industry, largely as a result of the growth of sponsorship, merchandising, endorsement of products and services, corporate hospitality and, above all, the sale and exploitation of broadcasting rights. New methods of exploiting sport content and new rules have been put in place. Yet, for all its prominence, television sport remains an under-research topic. To come to terms with this complex domain we need the kind of intellectual help and professional experience that Mike Milne offers us. He does that through a comprehensive, analytical account that is supported by solid documentary evidence and transparent argumentation.

One of the main strengths of the volume is the focus on the sports production sector. Drawing on his own personal experience working in the industry and a range of interviews with industry players, Milne offers insights into how macro level changes in sports broadcasting have shaped the supply side of the industry, namely sports programme production. A range of audiences, particularly in policy making, broadcasting industry, academia and sports federations, can benefit from this theoretical critical analysis and empirical national case studies.

Petros Iosifidis
Professor in Media Policy
City University London

Acknowledgements

With any project of this kind there are numerous people without whose help the finishing line would have remained tantalisingly in the distance. Early guidance came from Andrea Esser and Paul Rixon at Roehampton. Anthony McNicholas paved the way for my research to continue at the University of Westminster's Communication and Media Research Institute. Most gratitude and thanks goes to Jeannette Steemers. She showed remarkable patience as I found my way, then she challenged me to achieve the best outcome I could. The book would be much diminished without Jeanette's sharply focussed input. Over several years working in television sport numerous colleagues kindly gave their time to talk about many issues, shedding light on their areas of specialism and how much they thought 'the goalposts have moved'. I have tried to reflect their experience and concerns throughout as a key part of a missing supply-side account. Of course thanks, too, goes to Palgrave Macmillan for providing the chance for this text to reach a wider audience, it is an honour to be part of this prestigious series. The book attempts to shed light on aspects of television sport that are seldom seen and are often subject to acute commercial sensitivity. Every effort has been made to respect copyright and to provide accuracy throughout, so any material that ought to have been flagged for offside but has slipped through remains my responsibility.

Abbreviations and Acronyms

ABC	American Broadcasting Company
AFC	American Football Conference
AFL	American Football League
ATP	Association of Tennis Professionals
BBC	British Broadcasting Company
BSB	British Satellite Broadcasting
BSkyB	British Sky Broadcasting
CAT	Competition Appeals Tribunal
CBS	Columbia Broadcasting System
DCMS	Department of Culture, Media and Sport
EBU	European Broadcasting Union
EC	European Commission
ECB	England and Wales Cricket Board
EP	European Parliament
ESPN	Entertainment and Sports Programming Network
ETP	European Tour [of Golf] Productions
EU	European Union
F1	Formula 1
FA	The Football Association
FFP	Financial Fair Play [Rules]
FIFA	Fédération Internationale de Football Association
FinSyn	Financial Interest and Syndication Rules
HBO	Home Box Office
HBS	Host Broadcast Services
HD	High Definition
IAAF	International Association of Athletics Federations
IBA	Independent Broadcasting Authority
IBC	International Broadcast Centre
IMG	International Management Group
IOC	International Olympic Committee
IP	Intellectual Property
IRB	International Rugby Board
ISL	International Sport and Leisure
ITA	Independent Television Authority
ITC	Independent Television Commission
ITT	Invitation To Tender

ITV	Independent Television [Network]
MLB	Major League Baseball
MoTD	Match of The Day
MRO	Multilateral Running Order
NBA	National Basketball Association
NBC	National Broadcasting Company
NCAA	National Collegiate Athletic Association
NFC	National Football Conference
NFL	National Football League
NHL	National Hockey League
NTL	National Telecommunications Limited
OB	Outside Broadcast
OBS	Olympic Broadcasting Services
Ofcom	Independent regulator and competition authority for the UK communications industries.
OFT	Office of Fair Trading
OTAB	Olympic Television Archive Bureau
PL	Premier League
PLP	Premier League Productions
PPV	Pay Per View
PSB	Public Service Broadcaster
RF	Radio Frequency
RFP	Request For Production
RHB	Rights Holding Broadcaster
RPC	Restricted Practices Court
TBS	Turner Broadcasting System
Telco	Telecommunications Company
TOP	The Olympic Programme
TRIPS	Trade Related Property Rights
TSL	Television Sport and Leisure
TUPE	Transfer of Undertakings Regulations
TVWF	Television without Frontiers Directive
TWI	TransWorld International
UCL	UEFA Champions League
UEFA	Union of European Football Associations
UFC	Ultimate Fighting Championship
VOD	Video On Demand
VT	Video Tape
WIPO	World Intellectual Property Organisation
WTO	World Trade Organisation

1
Introduction

The rise of television sport

£5.14 billion: the value achieved in early 2015 by the Premier League as it sold domestic broadcasting rights in the UK for three years from 2016 to 2019. The Premier League is now the world's second most lucrative sports league; the NFL, by accessing the larger US domestic market, leads the way as it generates £4.5 billion each season. Looking at the overall market in 2015, Pricewaterhouse Coopers estimates global sports business, including all revenue streams, was worth $145 billion (PwC, 2015). The value of Premier League broadcasting rights is particularly remarkable because, as recently as 1986, no one in the UK wanted to broadcast league football, not even highlights. Transformations of this scale and magnitude do not happen by accident.

Even with an increase in mobile and online viewing this is an era when, for most people, watching sport means turning on the television rather than visiting a stadium to see an event. In summer 2012 the sheer amount of television sport broadcast reached a new high mark including, in the UK, the EURO 2012 football tournament, tennis from Queens and Wimbledon, Bradley Wiggins' success in the Tour de France, the London Olympics and the Paralympics. The ability of elite sport to attract very large audiences when broadcast on television, particularly on free-to-air television, underlines its continuing popularity. As a practical way for advertisers and sponsors to reach mass audiences, television sport has no equal. But scratch beneath the surface and a different picture emerges. Coverage of EURO 2012, the Tour de France, the London Olympics and Paralympics all came from federation-run broadcast operations aimed squarely at global audiences, leaving rights-holding broadcasters to concentrate on presentation for their local markets. In television sport things are not always as they first appear.

The transformation of television sport

Since the late 1980s the sector has been subject to unprecedented transformation as new methods and new rules have quietly been put in place. For all its prominence, television sport remains a surprisingly under-researched area. Like many, I have enjoyed watching television sport. But, as an executive producer, I have also worked on television sport in the UK, US and Japan, embracing sports as diverse as the NFL, NBA, MLB, Formula 1, World Rally Championships, Football Italia, Premier League, Bundesliga, Rugby Union and Sumo. Whilst my professional experience regularly placed me on the frontline, it was not enough for me to fully understand what has happened to television sport.

In terms of what we see, television sport consistently achieves remarkably high technical standards as it delivers captivating and sometimes spectacular engagement that can live long in our memory. But a nagging doubt remains: is this parade of slick technology and polished logistics a veneer that obscures our view of what is really happening? Thinking about what we see and where we see it, why has television sport in the UK changed beyond recognition in less than 25 years? Or, more generally, why does international sport coverage appear to have become more homogenised, even a bit bland? In an era that could have delivered unprecedented creativity, why are replication and inhibition recurrent themes? Even in a culture where hyperbole is the name of the game, is there really no place for *any* critical comment? This book is interested in who produces television sport, why it is produced the way it is and what the consequences might be.

Whilst there are several influential accounts – Holt (1989), Barnett (1990), Whannel (1992), Whitson (1998), Holt and Mason (2000), Boyle and Haynes (2000; 2004), Haynes (2005), Nauright and Schimmel (2005), Evens, Iosifidis and Smith (2013) – political economy interpretations of television sport remain at their best when painting the bigger picture. By focussing on major currents – for example, how the commodification of sport has accelerated (Mosco, 1996) as it is bound up in the processes of economic production and distribution (Mason, 1999) that deliver sport product on ever-increasing scales to international consumers (Nauright and Schimmel, 2005); the emergence of a sport-media-corporate axis (Falcous, 2005); or how sport is used as a battering ram to enter and take control of new markets (Herman and McChesney,

1997) – a demand side view has come to dominate discussion and has eclipsed a supply side interpretation. What is missing is an account of wider influences that trickle down and shape how television sports programmes are made, who makes them and what they finally look and sound like.

This book argues the transformation of television sport has been driven by a combination of interacting forces including broadcasting policy (media markets), technology, economics (broadcasting rights) and politics (media regulation). These forces mostly operate upstream and out of sight (i.e. before traditional production and distribution processes begin) and increasingly determine what sport we see, where we can see, and what the final output looks and sounds like.

In practice, developments in technology (encompassing transmission, production and distribution technology) are re-articulated via the broadcasting rights subsequently issued in the following cycle, typically every three years. The competition to acquire these broadcasting rights is mitigated (usually a further cycle behind) by industry regulators; these regulators and competition authorities echo the prevailing national or regional media policy.

A critical and often overlooked component is the *interplay* of technological development, broadcasting rights and regulation. As technological developments tend to move more quickly than rights or regulation,

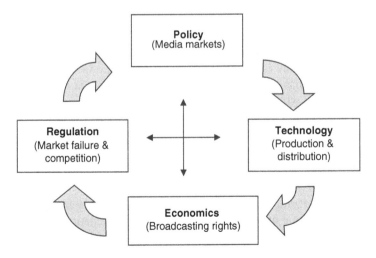

Figure 1.1 Policy, technology, economics and regulation

then regulators and competition authorities can be in a constant process of trying to catch up with developments. The book remains aware of (a) how economic markets work, (b) how market forces affect economic outcomes, and (c) how powerful actors attempt to manipulate market forces to advance their private interest (Gilpin, 2001:40).

Designed to complement the bigger picture usually provided by a political economy view, the objective here is to offer a convincing supply side perspective, one that tracks the impact of transformations downstream in the work of broadcasters, media providers, independent production companies as well as individual sports producers and directors. The book asks *how* television sport has changed, *why* it has changed so quickly and *what* these changes mean to practitioners and audiences.

The answers to three over-arching questions help to convey just how far the goalposts have been moved:

- Whilst sports and broadcasting systems in the US and UK started from diametrically opposed positions post-World War II, why have the similarities between them, including the adoption of a more overtly consumer-oriented approach in the UK, become the most noticeable features? How has the rise of global televised sports events and marketing-led television sport strategies accelerated this process?
- Transformations in television sports production since the mid-1990s have been driven by a combination of increasingly influential upstream forces including technology, sports broadcasting rights and regulation. How do these largely unseen pre-production processes influence what television sport looks and sounds like, where it can be seen and who can see it?
- What is the impact of pre-production processes on the downstream supply side, including (a) broadcasters (including *who* now provides sports media), (b) independent sports television production, and (c) the day-to-day work of sports producers and directors?

Specific consideration is also given to: 1) the remarkable growth in the volume and scope of television sport, 2) an unprecedented expansion in the number of channels and additional outlets, 3) fiercer competition between broadcasters and media providers to acquire elite sports broadcasting rights, including massive inflation in the cost of live broadcasting rights for the most popular sports, 4) the increasingly prescriptive demands on coverage required by federations, including the introduction of Production Manuals, 5) the introduction of federation-run host production operations and league-run channels that provide 'approved' coverage, 6) the increasing importance of presentation to local audiences by rights holding broadcasters and, 7) a growing emphasis on specialisation among sports producers and directors.

For Boyle and Haynes (2000:45), sport and television were 'two great cultural forms which simply proved to be irresistible to each other'. As a result, sport has come to matter a great deal to big businesses and to the managers of increasingly commercial and global media industries. Of particular interest is how, in a short period, English football reformulated its structure, ethos and governance to become aligned with the interests of corporate investment and the managerial tenets of advertising, marketing and public relations (Falcous, 2005). In 1992 the Premier League was formed turning league football into a private good consumed for profit in a fully-fledged market economy. A new era of sports broadcasting had arrived in the UK.

As economics became the primary measure of value, the formation of the Premier League reflects the activities of other leagues and federations. Around the world leagues and federations have exercised their market power to extend control over their events and subsequent television output, so an increasingly prescriptive approach to television sports production becomes apparent. This includes additional conditions that are written into sports broadcasting rights as they are issued which creates a degree of conformity across output, despite the current phase being defined by an ever-increasing volume of content. From around 2005, leagues and federations began to produce their own 'approved' television coverage of their signature events, including the Olympics and World Cup Finals. Federation-controlled *coverage* is aimed at global audiences; this leaves rights-holding national broadcasters to provide more localised *presentation* for their own markets. The split between coverage and presentation is a significant development. Sharing the idea of a strictly controlled brand image, the Premier League now produces and distributes its own television channel for international distribution outside the UK. With international broadcasting rights for 2013–16 in the region of £2 billion, then revenues for the next rights, 2016–19, are expected to set new records. Today, leagues and federations have much more to say in determining what sport we see, where we can see it and what the final output looks and sounds like.

The political economy of television sport

Given the symbiotic relationship between media and sports organisations, Evens, Iosifidis and Smith (2013:4) describe a political economy approach that addresses how the behaviour of media organisations is shaped by the economic and political context in which they operate. The backdrop is neoliberalism and how this view is promoted via its policies of privatisation, liberalisation of markets, deregulation (and re-regulation that promotes free-market competition), corporatisation and the withdrawal of the state from many areas of social provision. Who gets what, when and how are questions that are seldom asked by economists but are central issues in a political economy interpretation.

With the increasing marketisation of broadcasting, and with sport (particularly in the UK) shedding many of its cultural and social connections in conditions where economic value has come to reign supreme, so a political economy interpretation can help reveal currents that are, on first inspection, more elusive. This approach is used to interpret upstream transformations and to track the shifting relationships (and behaviours) that increasingly define televised sport. In *A Brief History of Neoliberalism*, Harvey (2005) describes 'accumulation through dispossession' (2005:159) and how neoliberalisation has meant the 'financialisation of everything' (2005:33). Although directed at wider developments, these ideas are apposite when discussing the trajectory of television sport. However, this interpretation extends the vertical value chain for television sport upstream and downstream to include: (a) the pivotal role of sports leagues and federations in determining final television output, and (b) a micro-level analysis of downstream activities, or the day-to-day workplace methods that illustrate the 'trickle down' effect of wider transformations. This view is very closely connected to current industry practice.

A central issue in the book is the role of intellectual property rights and how control of sport broadcasting rights has become a vital activity of broadcasters and media providers, one that often defines their identity. Haynes (2005:5) points out that 'to understand how copyright and other laws to protect intellectual property rights achieve their purpose, it is crucial to understand how different aspects of the media industry operate as technologies and businesses...' The book considers how sport has become so important to broadcasters and media providers. It updates understanding by examining the conditions that have transformed television sport and it offers new access to the relatively closed media world of television sport. A thorough discussion of the transformation of television sport should address league and federation behaviour in more detail, including sports economics. This is a surprising omission from most political economy accounts. Sport is a sector where many economic rules appear to be inverted, particularly issues related to monopoly behaviour, including single entity co-operation (i.e. organising competitions) and joint venture co-operation (collective sale of broadcasting rights). The essence of sports economics is captured by Neale (1964:14): 'It is clear that professional sports are a natural monopoly, marked by definite peculiarities both in the structure and in the functioning of their markets'. Considering several factors, including (a) elite athletic performance, (b) the shared experience that sport provides, (c) the uncertainty of outcome for live events, (d) lack of an adequate substitute in other programme forms, and (e) with demand from media providers to acquire rights for the most popular sports outstripping supply, then scarcity is said to exist. When scarcity exists 'demand theory' says that rationing devices must be chosen and the most prominent device is price, consequently the value of sports broadcasting rights rise as a result of competition from broadcasters and media providers. Scarcity, rationing and competition [for sports broadcasting rights] represent an 'economic trinity', Fort (2006:15).

Economically, the revenue side of professional sport changed forever with the willingness of advertisers to pay to access audiences that watch sports programming and the crucial importance of revenue from broadcasting rights was established, argues Fort (2006:53). How leagues and federations acquired significant market power, often via cartel control of broadcasting rights, is mapped.

A complementary interpretation would also benefit from extending discussion of media economics, including examination of the vertical value chain in television production. A fundamental issue for media providers is how to collect value from the audiences its programmes and schedules attract. For Picard (1989:17–19) media firms operate in a 'dual product' market. The two commodities generated are: 1) content (programmes produced or acquired and subsequently broadcast in recognisable schedules and; 2) the audiences that choose to watch. Commercial television networks can price and sell access to their audiences to advertisers and sponsors and the retention of audiences is critical to all broadcasters, including Public Service Broadcasters (PSBs).

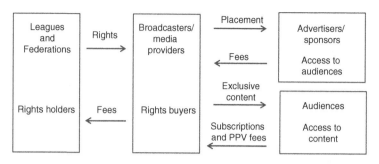

Figure 1.2   Willingness to pay in sports broadcasting rights

The ability of popular sports to consistently deliver audiences with more efficiency and demographic accuracy than many other genres is critical. Dominated by a small number of large firms television sports broadcasting is an oligopolistic market, where the activities of one actor can have a significant impact on others; it is a market where economies of scale and scope can provide a competitive edge. Looking at individual media providers, Doyle (2002) uses vertical deconstruction to reveal a basic range of functions. These functions start upstream with (a) the creation (or acquisition) of intellectual property rights and work through succeeding downstream stages, including (b) the production of programmes, and (c) the distribution (transmission) of content and services to the audience.

Developments in technology also allow media providers to collect value directly from audiences by means of subscriptions and pay-per-view services. Media firms can approach these basic functions differently depending on how they are funded, including 1) commercial free-to-air terrestrial broadcasters, 2) free-to-air terrestrial PSB broadcasters, 3) free-to-air commercial PSB broadcasters, 4) pay television services, including satellite, cable and internet providers and, 5) further pay

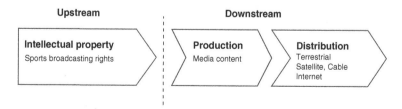

Figure 1.3   Vertical supply chain

content media services often via online or mobile platforms. The role of independent sports production companies is also of interest as these firms seldom hold broadcasting rights or have direct access to audiences themselves.

Objectives and outline

By asking three over-arching questions, the book examines fundamental changes to the television sport supply chain; it provides a bridge between increasingly influential upstream activities (technology, broadcasting rights and regulation) before zooming in to examine the downstream impact of transformations on broadcasters, media providers, independent sports, independent production companies and the day-to-day work of producers and directors, the final intermediaries. There are two objectives: 1) to demonstrate the sheer scale of transformation that has taken place and 2) to identify a range of consequences, including the extent of league and federation control over television sport output, the split between coverage and presentation, and the pressure placed on independent production companies, producers and directors to specialise. Bringing these developments to light will serve further discussion.

Chapter 2 begins by addressing a surprising gap in the political economy interpretation of television sport, as a comparison of technological, economic and political developments in the US and UK since 1945 is provided. The combination of professional sport and commercial television found in the US contrasted acutely with conditions in the UK dominated by amateur sport and a public service broadcaster operating in a monopoly. After a prolonged period of resistance, how the UK came to adopt a more consumer-oriented approach typically seen in the US and, in some instances, has become even more overtly commercial in outlook says a lot about the state of play today. Chapter 2 considers the incursion of marketing and promotional strategies (Giulianotti, 1999; 2005), how new types of corporate integration have been adopted (Whitson, 1998; Falcous, 2005) and the extension of transnational capitalism into sports (Nauright and Schimmel, 2005). Examples cited include the rise of the Olympics, World Cup Finals, the NBA and the UEFA Champions League.

An analysis of how forces operating upstream increasingly shape television sport is set out in chapters 3, 4 and 5. The ways technology, broadcasting rights (economics) and regulation (politics) are closely interconnected and how, *working together*, they exert a significant influence on television sport is unpacked.

Todreas (1999) identifies three phases since 1992 including: (1) the limits of linear analogue technology, (2) the transition from tape-based media to digital media, and (3) high definition and beyond. Chapter 3 expands understanding with: (a) an overview of transmission technology as an important forerunner in the switch to digital, (b) by examining the limits of analogue technology in sports production, (c) identifying pivotal developments in digital technology, (d) comparing analogue and digital workflows to illustrate the sheer scale of transformation, and (e) reviewing the extraordinary increase in volume and scope of content that can be produced rapidly in a digital workplace. Technological determinism is avoided and a political economy perspective is added by asking *who* does *what* and *why*, with the Premier League providing a case study.

Transformations in technology are closely linked to developments in broadcasting rights. Rights tend to follow one cycle behind technological developments and include important new ways of distributing content plus the emergence of new markets, including overseas markets. Chapter 4 tackles sports broadcasting rights by considering: (a) what is copyright and intellectual property and how this is connected to the market (b) the changing values and definitions of sports broadcasting rights, and (c) the implications of rights for producers, with a case study from the UEFA Champions League. How prescriptive conditions are frequently added to broadcasting rights by leagues and federations, reinforcing their dominant position, is a critical development.

Chapter 5 focuses on the role of regulation from (a) national and international level broadcasting policies such as the list of protected events, (b) examples of intervention directed at the Premier League and the UEFA Champions League, (c) the regulation of both markets *and* content in the UK, and (d) the widening gap between regulatory intention and actual output as seen in regional production quotas and the application of the Transfer of Undertakings (Protection of Employment) Regulations (TUPE). Together chapters 3, 4 and 5 explain how influential decisions have migrated upstream, away from broadcasters towards leagues and federations, and so extends the work of Todreas (1999), Doyle (2002) and Gratton and Solberg (2007). The ways that broadcasters and producers engage with technology, broadcasting rights and regulation is framed from several angles.

Chapters 6 and 7 offer insights on a micro level as the trickle-down effect of wider transformations are identified. As demand continues to outstrip supply, increased competition to acquire sports broadcasting rights has delivered good economic news for the elite leagues and federations (Fort, 2006:53). But what are the challenges now faced by broadcasters and media providers?

Chapter 6 considers a range of challenges now faced by broadcasters and media providers including: (a) the difficulties of evaluating broadcasting rights values in competitive markets where the commercial performance of broadcasters and media providers has become increasingly linked to the acquisition and retention of critical sports broadcasting rights, an activity that also reshapes the downstream market for content provision; (b) the rise of federation-based *coverage* of major sports events, (c) the subsequent importance of local *presentation* in sports television and, (d) despite the substantially increased volume and scope of content, how there is a marked *reduction* in critical content.

Chapter 7 identifies important trends in independent sports production. Ownership of independent sports production companies by private equity firms or by other investors provides an economic paradigm shift that is used to explain the emergence and rapid extension of new roles on the production side, including legal, business and production management positions. The extent to which the operational side of production has become separated from the editorial and creative side, including the rise of production management departments, is examined. Also under scrutiny is the different ways that content is commissioned and the consequences for independent production companies. With tension between prescription and creativity growing, how is the work of individual producers and directors being recast, including the need to specialise?

Chapter 8 provides the conclusion as it reprises key developments in the shift of market power from broadcasters and media providers to the leagues and federations that sell broadcasting rights. In the race between money and meaning there was only likely to be one winner, commercial values and the market are the driving forces in the digital era of television sport. But this new era presents a paradox. Afraid to bite the hand that feeds, has television sport become a place where broadcasters, media providers, independent sports production companies, and individual producers and directors have exciting new methods at their disposal, but they also have to play by the new rules set by the leagues and federations?

For the record, and reflecting the current climate, all the contributors and practitioners interviewed in the book did so under conditions of strict confidentiality and anonymity. Many people kindly gave their time and provided long form interviews that covered a wide range of topics, while others responded positively to short form interviews that often came out of workplace activities – their contributions are crucial to the book and were received with appreciation and thanks. However, it should also be noted that several other specialists did initially offer to take part but, later, chose not to do so. Speaking to producers and executives closely linked to federation-based activities often drew a blank, as, even with anonymity, some were unwilling to participate.

2
History

A surprising omission in the political economy interpretation of television sports is a comparison of technological, economic and political developments in the US and UK between 1945 and 1995. With researchers considering a range of topics – from the incursion of marketing and promotional strategies (Giulianotti, 1999, 2005), how new types of corporate integration have been adopted (Whitson, 1998; Falcous, 2005) and the extension of transnational capitalism into sports (Nauright and Schimmel, 2005) – Boyle and Haynes (2000:66) view development in the UK as reflecting 'a mode of organisation that is more akin to the long-standing consumer-orientated configuration of sport in North America'. This is surprising because, for long periods, change was resisted in Britain, the subsequent speed at which overt commercialism and a more consumer-oriented approach was adopted is fascinating and a distinguishing feature between 1970 and 1995. In many ways the Premier League now demonstrates unprecedented levels of corporate behaviour and commodification that surpasses practice in US Major Leagues, long regarded as providing a benchmark. This chapter charts how, despite some remarkable differences, the UK has gravitated towards practices found in the US.

Post-World War II, the relationships between sport and television in the US and UK could hardly have been further apart; the combination of professional sport and commercial, entertainment-driven, free-to-air network television in the US contrasted starkly with the UK where there was an amateur ethos and paternalistic management of sport allied to a public service broadcast monopoly. Focussing on the NFL and English league football, the development of sports television through to 1970 is reviewed.

The next section tracks the technological, economic (particularly the rising value of sports broadcasting rights) and political development trajectories in the US and UK as free-market principles and commercialism became prevalent between 1970 and 1995. In conclusion, it is argued that by the early 1990s it had become the similarities rather than the differences in the ways that sport and television function in the US and the UK that stood out.

But something else was happening. Just how key attitudes attached to sport have radically changed in only 36 years can be seen in the transformation of the Olympics, from 1948 and the British Government-backed post-War London austerity games, to 1984 and the aggressively commercial, privately financed, free-market funded model pioneered in Los Angeles. The impact of the 1984 Los Angeles Games sport-television-corporate model and the dramatic rise of global televised sports events are considered. The underlying theme is how market power has migrated from the broadcasters, moving upstream to the leagues and federations. This is important background context for subsequent discussion about how non-controversial international television coverage is now provided directly by the federations – tracking this significant development is essential to understanding just how much television sport has been transformed.

2.1 Sport and television in United States and UK 1945 to 1970

US Sport, open professionalism

Pure amateurism simply never existed in the US, argues Pope (1997). When baseball established itself in the 1870s as an entertainment business run by its owners, boards of directors and non-playing managers it was already openly professional. The very idea of sport as entertainment, or as a business, did not cause the sort of apoplexy it did in Britain. The four major US sports leagues are: Major League Baseball (MLB), the National Football League (NFL), the National Basketball Association (NBA) and the National Hockey League (NHL). Even though Major League Baseball (MLB) was a lucrative business for its owners it remained, from a legal point of view at least, defined as a game. MLB also had the good fortune to be formed prior to the 1880 Sherman Antitrust Act that banned monopolies, so it was exempt from potential legal action. In other words, sport in the US was not regarded as trade in the traditional sense and leagues, like the MLB, were subsequently free to engage in cartel behaviour (Fort, 2006:261; Pope, 1997:65).

This important idea had a profound impact on US sports' relationship with television; from the outset sport, entertainment and business were closely linked in the pursuit of profit.

US television, advertiser-funded commercial broadcasting

In some countries broadcasting was considered too important to be left to commercial exploitation; the US was not one of them. By using formidable political leverage large corporations seized control of the US broadcasting industry before a public service system could be established (Herman and McChesney, 1997:14). These corporations had recognised the commercial potential of radio as an advertising-funded medium; the post-World War II US television boom was funded by advertising. Advertising is central to the US free-to-air terrestrial broadcast networks because the economic forces favouring mass consumption of media is reinforced by the simultaneous production of audiences for sale to advertisers (Owen and Wildman, 1992:151; Picard, 1989). The viability of the free-to-air broadcast networks rests in their ability to remain the most convenient route for advertisers to reach mass audiences. The sheer scale of the US market is a key point of difference compared to the smaller UK market.

There are consequences for relying on advertising to fund network television. Principally it is the value that advertisers place on the audience, rather than audience preferences that determines which programmes are provided. In this system the broadcaster has an incentive to maximise the supply of programmes that attract the audiences that advertisers will pay to reach – a review of programme supply models can be found in Owen and Wildman (1992). As the US networks sought to correlate their advertising revenues with the ability to attract audiences, a preference developed for programmes that appeared at the same time each week. Programmes with familiar characters and storylines that were developed in only slightly varied situations and that carried over narratives from previous episodes were considered to generate viewer loyalty. According to Jay (2004:91) sports coverage fitted very neatly into this emerging pattern. As much as 30% of the prime-time schedule was devoted to sports coverage, making it a crucial part of early television programming in the US.

US television and sport

In just 8 years, between 1948 and 1956, the percentage of American homes that had television jumped from 3% to 81%, (Jay, 2004:61).

The arrival of television had several important consequences for sports including:

- The relocation of existing teams. This was the *viable threat* of moving a team to more lucrative media-markets created by new demographic shifts. From the mid-1950s teams began to move, including the Boston Braves to Milwaukee in 1953, then to Atlanta in 1965; in 1957 the Brooklyn Dodgers and New York Giants moved to Los Angeles and San Francisco respectively.
- The rapid expansion of professional sports leagues and the creation of new teams.
- The development of new leagues that challenged the monopoly of the existing order. The American Football League (AFL) was established in 1960 to challenge the NFL, baseball's Continental League forced the American League to admit two new teams in 1961, and in basketball the American Basketball Association (ABA) was formed in 1967 to challenge the NBA.

The location of a team or composition of a league was heavily influenced early on by the revenue that teams received from selling their broadcasting rights. Advertisers were attracted to the audiences that televised sports drew and were willing to pay networks for access to these audiences. Initially this was in the form of sponsorship. Gillette often sponsored the entire cost of a sports programme, supplying the networks with sufficient funds to pay the professional sports leagues for broadcasting rights (Jay, 2004:102). In 1947 Gillette paid $175,000 to attach its name to television coverage of the baseball World Series on NBC. Also attracted to the narratives of the emerging televised-sports marketplace, beer manufacturers established associations between consumer products and sport. Single company sponsorship of televised sports events continued throughout much of the 1950s. The mutual relationship between professional sport, entertainment, business and television was the American way writ large.

UK Sport, paternalistic amateurism

The historic hostility to commercialism among British sports ruling bodies is indisputable: 'the rule of amateurs kept capitalism at bay in British sport' states Holt (1989:281). The roots of paternalistic amateurism lie in the Victorians' organising genius for games. It was the British who invented many modern sports, codified their rules and exported them to the world, e.g. association football, rugby union and rugby league, cricket, tennis and golf. Perelman (2012) links the origins of modern sport in England with the capitalist mode of production and the consolidation of imperialism. For the British, sportsmanship was the foundation stone. It was not so much *what* the British played, as the *way* that they played it that mattered most. Teams had very strong social and geographical links that went a long way to defining their identity. Post-World War II the idea that sport might be an industry or a form of commercial entertainment would not have been acceptable to its managers who, themselves, were also amateurs. The FA in particular, as Conn (1997) points out, worked hard to protect football from 'the corrosive idea that it [football] was purely entertainment, a business purely about money...The FA even had rules against directors making money out of clubs' (Conn, 1997:169). For most of the second half of the twentieth century British sport was poised between a rather idealised amateur past and a commercialised free-market future (Holt and Mason, 2000). In terms of a battle, this was to prove a mismatch.

The decline of amateurism in the UK

Although amateurism remained popular in the 1950s it was soon in decline. Whilst Macmillan's Britain was a very different place from Eisenhower's America, the late 1950s and 1960s were still largely prosperous years that prompted Macmillan's famous claim of 1957 that 'Britons had never had it so good'. Football, boxing, golf, horse racing, cycling and cricket were promising sports for budding professionals and, from the 1960s, amateurism began to lose its appeal. Contributory factors included the growth in international competition, changing expectations of what constituted success, greater prosperity, and increased leisure options. The idea that sport was something to which financial value should *not* be attached began to seem rather out-dated. By the 1970s being an amateur came to mean little more than taking part. For Holt and Mason (2000), it was the market power of sports performers whose television appearances attracted the interest of advertisers and sponsors that triggered the demise of the amateur ethic.

Of all Britain's sports organisations it was football that claimed cultural centrality. The post-World War II repositioning of football signals the start of a general transformation in British sport. But sport on British television was valued very differently than in the US.

BBC Television and sport

In the UK a public service broadcasting system (PSB) was adopted to address basic market failure, funding is provided via a license fee. The

BBC, argue Curran and Seaton (2003), was founded on a rejection of market forces and politics insofar as the British government considered that broadcasting demanded a new form of administration with social and not financial priorities. The BBC was set up as a vertically integrated programme maker, channel provider and broadcast distributor (Szymanski, 2006). Owen and Wildman (1992) note that there is a sharp distinction between the behaviour of a monopolist, as is the case with the BBC, and the behaviour of a competitive industry. As was the case with the US networks BBC Television placed a great emphasis on broadcasting sport, but for quite different reasons. Re-iterating, Whannel (1992), Gratton and Solberg (2007) argue it made economic sense as, post-World War II, the BBC benefited from an enormous inequality in market power between the buyers (the monopoly broadcaster BBC) and the sellers of broadcasting rights (the amateur sports organisations). An annual calendar of broadcast events – one that resonated with the winter and summer seasons of sport – had already been created on BBC radio as early as the 1930s (Scannell and Cardiff, 1991) so delivering important sporting events to a national audience became a cornerstone of the BBC's PSB remit (Boyle and Haynes, 2000:69). As viewers joined the shared experience of BBC Television coverage, these events came to reinforce popular ideas about being British, even though the choice of events had a tendency to reflect the tastes of BBC managers. Arguing that it was promoting events to a national audience, the BBC resisted the payment of broadcasting rights fees to sport. BBC Television's first major sports broadcast came from the 1948 London Olympics, but it wasn't until the 1950s that broadcasting attained any sort of momentum as previously modest sales of television sets were boosted in 1953 by coverage of the Coronation.

The BBC's monopoly ended when Independent Television (ITV) was approved as part of the Television Act of 1954. Around the same time the era of sports broadcasting rights formally arrived in the UK. Copyright issues had led to a restriction of television access to sport in the UK. Significantly, the Labour government's Committee on Copyrights (1952) announced that rights to television sports performances should be vested in the broadcaster on agreement of remuneration to sports promoters for any loss of revenue incurred. The BBC paid £1000 to broadcast the 1953 FA Cup Final with Stanley Matthews. The BBC's head of Outside broadcasts, Gerald Cock writing in the Radio Times, said 'It is a dismal prospect when the governing body of a sport originated and built up and entirely supported by amateurs, should be captured by professionals whose interest apparently is commercial' (Cock, 1930). Sports governing bodies remained wary of the potential threat to attendances that television coverage might cause; such concerns kept coverage of live league football off British television screens until the early 1980s. In the UK, the staple diet of sport on television was edited highlights in a magazine format with live presentation links, like *Grandstand*. The BBC's Saturday afternoon sports magazine debuted in 1958 and ran until January 2007, almost forty years.

Value and the monopoly provision of sport

Meanwhile, in the US, sport was changing television. As the cost of single company sponsorship of sports events rose sharply in the 1960s the networks started selling advertising spots to multiple companies, essentially the style of commercial breaks we see today. Advertisers were able to buy access to network television audiences in a number of ways, with as much as 80% of time committed in the up-front market, where segments are sold centrally by the networks on behalf of their affiliate stations. Owen and Wildman (1992) note three types of non-network television advertising: barter-syndication (where advertising time is bundled together with programming and sold as a package), the national spot market (where time is purchased in local markets and therefore bypasses the networks altogether) and, from the 1980s, advertising sold on cable channels. The ability to make an immediate impact by attracting massive audiences, for example by broadcasting the most popular sports, came to command a special value for broadcasters and advertisers. As values began to rise, sports governing bodies adopted cartel behaviour to monopolise the provision of their sport to media providers.

Ironically, it was amateur college sports that broke new ground. From 1949 college sport commanded significant fees for its broadcasting rights when CBS paid $100,000 for the rights to the annual Rose Bowl game from Pasadena, CA, (Jay, 2004:99). In 1952 the Television Plan allowed the National Collegiate Athletic Association (NCAA) to negotiate the broadcasting rights collectively for all Division 1A college football.

Whilst the NCAA led the way, the turning point in the relationship between professional sports and media providers came in the mid-1950s when team owners decided to establish the NFL as a single economic cartel with a monopoly provision of the sport to the television networks. By 1967 the NFL and AFL champion teams – still playing in parallel leagues – faced each other in a showdown game designed specifically for television that quickly became American sports' most spectacular annual event – the *SuperBowl*. The cost of advertising slots within *SuperBowl* broadcasts and the transmission of bespoke advertising campaigns became a cult television event in itself and one that continues today. On the back of television exposure, by 1969 professional football (NFL) had taken over from baseball (MLB) as America's national game. The rising popularity of the NFL on television delivered important target demographics to advertisers. Media providers collected this value (the rates they charged advertisers for slot fees) and passed it through to the NFL in the form of sports broadcasting rights fees (Fort, 2006:84). The correlation between the advertising revenue a televised sport can attract and the value of its broadcasting rights was established and remains a viable measure of value in many markets today.

Sports broadcasting rights in the United States

During the 1960s the market for sports broadcasting rights in the US was changed by four factors described by McChesney (1989):

1) For the first time television was available in most American homes.
2) The technology of sports broadcasting was improving with slow motion and colour pictures increasing the quality of the viewing experience.
3) The Sports Broadcasting Act of 1961 allowed professional teams to negotiate together as a cartel with broadcasters and so substantially increased their market power.
4) Media providers recognised the potential attraction of sports broadcasting to advertisers; this audience demographic was attractive to advertisers and a premium for those slots could be charged.

As competition among broadcasters to capture the most popular sports broadcasting rights increased the result was scarcity. As the value of rights began to escalate market power migrated from broadcasters to the leagues. As noted, the NCAA was the first sports organisation to adopt cartel behaviour and from 1949, in a single decade, the price of broadcasting rights to NCAA college football increased almost 450% from $1.14 million, to $5.1 million as CBS and NBC, now joined by ABC, raised their bids in successive contracts.

The 1964 Tokyo Olympics is mentioned anecdotally as the turning point for a general upward spiral in sports broadcasting rights fees. However, there was an increase in competition for rights as the market adjusted from a duopoly to an oligopoly with the arrival of an ambitious and sports-oriented ABC. Whilst CBS acquired broadcasting rights to the 1960 Rome Olympics, it was ABC that won the rights for the 1964

Tokyo Olympics. Collated from various sources, the rights fees paid for subsequent summer Olympics were:

Table 2.1   Summer Olympics, US broadcasting rights fees

Date	Network	Rights fees $
1960	CBS	$394,000
1964	ABC	$1.5 million
1968	ABC	$4.5 million
1972	ABC	$7.5 million
1976	ABC	$25 million
1980	NBC	$87 million
1984	ABC	$225 million

Sources: Collated from Kay (2004), Fernandez (2009), Stanford (2010).

Although the cost of broadcasting rights to the Olympics continued to rise, it can be argued that the burgeoning relationship between the NFL and television was more significant. In 1958, a game between the Baltimore Colts and the New York Giants is credited with transforming the NFL into a major consumer product. Seen live on television by an audience estimated to be anywhere between 30 and 45 million, the first sudden-death overtime championship game climaxed in a glorious finale for the Colts. For many fans, this game was the greatest ever played. Two years later, in 1960, the formation of the rival American Football League (AFL) demonstrated the growing importance of television to sports and vice versa. Whilst the AFL lost $3 million in its first year of operation, in 1964 NBC offered a $36 million contract for five years coverage, around $7.2 million per season and a substantial fee paid not for the original NFL but for a rival league. According to Jay (2004) NBC's bid came after CBS had offered the NFL $14 million for the rights to broadcast games for two years. Between 1961 and 1963 ratings for football on both networks had risen by 50%, apparently justifying such strong investment. On January 15 1967, the first SuperBowl game was played. According to Gratton and Solberg (2007:70) between 1967 and 2005 the average cost of a SuperBowl advertisement soared by more than 6,000%, which is 12 times the rate of the average network prime time's inflation in advertising cost over the same period. During the 1960s NFL Commissioner, Pete Rozelle, realised the power of consolidation and the need for competitive balance between the league's teams. He created a new business model for American football, ultimately making the NFL far more financially valuable than other American professional league sports, even though it had far fewer games per season to offer to television. Whilst the NFL continued to set the benchmark for the remarkable revenues it collected from the sale of broadcasting rights it should be remembered that broadcasters were, essentially, making massive bets on their ability to make a profit by selling access to large audiences to advertisers by televising sport.

Sports broadcasting rights in the UK

The impact of increased competition among broadcasters in the UK did *not* lead to a dramatic increase in the cost of acquiring broadcasting rights to sport as it had done in the US. Instead the BBC and ITV came to act as an informal cartel in suppressing the fees they paid for sports broadcasting rights. This practice lasted through to the mid-1970s. However, in the mid-1950s, parliamentary debate centred on whether or not there should be a free market in sporting events at all, or if the activity of commercial television in acquiring sports broadcasting rights should be strictly regulated. In 1956 government intervention came in the form of a national list of protected sports events. The listed events were considered to be of major importance to society and, consequently, they should be made available to as many television viewers as possible on free-to-air television. According to the Department for Culture, Media and Sport (DCMS) the original list was the result of a voluntary agreement between the BBC and ITV, (DCMS, 2009). The list consisted of the FA Cup Final, Wimbledon, England Test Matches, the Derby, the Grand National, the Boat Race and the Olympics and Commonwealth games when held in the UK. When BBC Two launched in 1964, it gave the corporation the option to switch sports broadcasting between its channels therefore guaranteeing continued coverage in the case of an event over-running its planned duration; this became a useful negotiating tool. Neither the reallocation of ITV franchises in 1967, nor the arrival of Channel Four in 1982 had a significant impact on the prevailing BBC/ITV duopoly and the ability to acquire rights to the most popular sports at very favourable rates – by 1970 the BBC was only paying £120,000 per season for rights to show the football league on their popular *Match of The Day* highlights presentation. In contrast to developments in the US, market power remained very firmly with the BBC and ITV and did not migrate upstream to the sports organisations.

For Boyle and Haynes (2000:38) a history of sport in the twentieth century is often presented as a history of televising sport. They also identify sport and the media as two great forces of the twentieth century, forces that 'have become entwined in a global business relationship, which brings both pain and pleasure to many and increasingly generates profit for a select few'. By the end of the 1960s many sports in the UK were facing a contested future, being pulled in one direction by increasingly out-dated amateur values and organisational structures and, in a new direction, by the influence of market forces and the lure of increased revenues via sponsorship and television exposure. British sport began for the first time to embrace commercialism. Whilst the process was usually cautious and gradual (Holt, 1989:354), the pace was beginning to quicken. The 1970s saw a new relationship develop between sport, television and sponsorship.

2.2 Free-markets, commercialism, sport and television in United States and UK 1970 to 1995

Between 1970 and the mid-1990s the television business was transformed as restrictive regulations were lifted in the US and UK. The technology of television production and of broadcast/distribution was revolutionised as a multitude of broadcasting platforms, some controlled by new owners, challenged the existing broadcasting order. With increased competition to acquire attractive content, the relationship between sport and television changed forever – the willingness to pay of advertisers, sponsors and viewers became an increasingly important factor. In the US, the value of broadcasting rights to the most popular sports, like the NFL, began to rise dramatically in the 1970s followed by a further escalation in the 1980s. Although the value of broadcasting rights had been repressed in the UK these also began to rise quickly in the late 1980s, as competition to acquire live football rights gained momentum. By the 1990s it can be argued that the Premier League had created a more overtly commercial and corporate structure than its counterparts in the US and was more profit-driven than any other professional sport before, including the NFL. These unprecedented changes and the economic consequences for sports broadcasting rights in the US and UK are now reviewed.

The rise of the NFL

The political foundations of the established networks' protected position began to unravel in the early 1970s. Among the consequences the broadcast networks turned more of their attention towards producing in-house sports and news programmes, activities that were not restricted by regulation policy to the extent that entertainment series were. The rise in popularity of the NFL on US network television during the 1970s is, at least in part, a consequence of broadcasting deregulation and the Financial Interest and Syndication (*FinSyn*) rules that restricted in-house production of network prime-time entertainment series and option terms for syndication rights (Owen and Wildman, 1992).

The mid-1970s also saw increased competition among US media providers with the arrival of Ted Turner's, Turner Broadcast (TBS) in 1976 and in 1979 Bill Rasmussen launched the 24-hour-a-day cable sports broadcaster ESPN. This signalled an important shift in the relationship between sports and television in the US, for example:

- There was an immediate increase in the demand for broadcasting rights to fill longer on-air schedules.
- The established terrestrial broadcasting paradigm was altered by the addition of new delivery platforms that bypassed the existing networks and their advertising sales divisions.
- Cable provided a technological solution to long-term market failure insofar as it introduced a means of charging and collecting revenue directly from customers via subscriptions. In economic terms, the willingness-to-pay of cable customers could exceed the willingness-to-pay of advertisers.

Against this backdrop – and with new US subscription-based channels often regarded as a *supplement* rather than a full competitor to terrestrial free-to-air channels in the US (Gratton and Solberg, 2007) – the 1970s was a golden decade for the NFL, its popularity grew steadily and advertisers and sponsors sought access to the large audiences live televised coverage of NFL games drew. The NFL was the first professional sports league to fully recognise and collect this value. Revenue from broadcasting rights soon overtook revenue from sponsorship (of events, teams and venues), ticket revenues and merchandising. For Fort (2006), it is the willingness of advertisers and sponsors to pay to access television audiences that altered the revenue side of professional sports forever. In a sense the NFL remains a voluntary organisation; it is an unincorporated association, which means that no single corporation is able to own any of the 32 franchises. The teams, by acting collectively through the league and by adopting cartel behaviour, gained market power through monopoly control of media access to their own broadcasting rights.

It was Rottenberg (1956) who identified that the maintenance of competitive balance was fundamental to the economics of team sports and it was the NFL Commissioner, Pete Rozelle, who put this concept into practice. Recognising the power of consolidation among teams operating in strong geographic markets (in territories that were protected from competition through the league), Rozelle was able to create a league-wide equilibrium that made *every* NFL game potentially exciting to watch (Jay, 2004). As explained by Fort (2006), an uncertainty of outcome must be preserved in games for fans to care and maintain their interest and that means there must be some overall balance of competition between teams. The NFL came up with a range of mechanisms to achieve consistent competitive balance and, consequently, was able to enhance the value of its broadcasting rights. Among the mechanisms are (a) salary cap agreements, (b) a reverse-order-of-finish draft system for players entering the league, and (c) an equal share of broadcasting revenues. With fewer teams and, therefore, less games played across a season to sell (a 17 week regular season followed by play-off elimination rounds featuring 12 teams), the major networks competed to acquire scarce broadcasting rights to the NFL and so the value increased substantially with each new contract. It was a seller's market. For 1970 Gratton and Solberg (2007) cite the NFL as earning $49 million a year from CBS (for NFC games) and NBC (for AFC games), both contracts were for four years. ABC contributed $8.5 million for the rights to broadcast the newly created schedule of Monday night games. By contrast, in 1970 the BBC paid £120,000 for the rights to show highlights from the Football League. Also of note: whilst NFL rights were split (or rationed) between the (then) 3 major networks, the copyright to all NFL broadcast material resided with the league and *not* with the networks that produced the coverage.

Increased competition among US broadcasters

The arrival of viable competition to the terrestrial free-to-air broadcasters increased the relative scarcity of broadcasting rights for the most popular sports driving up values, but what was different was the degree of inflation in the 1980s. Despite the increased competition from new media providers including pay-TV channels, a competitive edge was retained by the free-to-air networks because, as Jay (2004) reminds us, television sport is a medium for renting audiences to advertisers so the ability to deliver very large audiences combined with frequent breaks in play was a compelling proposition. This helps explain why, in contrast to the UK, Major League sports in the US have retained a strong presence on the free-to-air terrestrial broadcast networks, resisting the temptation to migrate wholesale to subscription-based television networks (Szymanski, 2006: Evens, Iosifidis and Smith, 2013). Illustrating this point, News Corporation purchased the Fox Broadcasting Company in 1985 and developed it into the fourth free-to-air independent tele-vision system, building on the existing network to compete with the three major US networks. FOX Sports was set up in 1994 following the acquisition of broadcasting rights to NFC games for four years (the NFC has teams in most of the largest US markets, including New York, Washington, Philadelphia, Chicago and San Francisco) with FOX pay-ing $1.58 billion to strip CBS of the rights. Significantly, FOX Sports, a sister corporation to BSkyB, was *not* set up as a stand-alone subscription-based service or even as a direct broadcast satellite television service in the mould of BSkyB even though, like BSkyB, it was transformed by the acquisition of exclusive live broadcasting rights.

It has been argued that US sport is less troubled when being described as a commodity, or as a business designed to generate profit. In another distinction from practices in the UK and Europe, the US Major Leagues were very much attuned to the needs of television from the outset. Con-sequently, the boundaries between what suited television coverage and what was enshrined in the rules of the game remained flexible and open to review. For example, the two-minute time-out at the end of each half in NFL games is widely attributed to the need for a premium advertising break as the action mounted. Today, teams are allowed to challenge on-field refereeing decisions via a video replay seen by audiences at home and for which they are charged a time-out. In the case of the NBA, inno-vations originally provided to enhance television coverage have become signature parts of the game, including the three-point shot and the 24-second shot clock introduced in 1954 to encourage faster play.

Leagues apart

Between the 1970s and mid-1980s the contrast between English league football and the NFL could not have been greater, if anything they were even further apart than they had been in 1945. Whilst the protected list regulations and the BBC/ITV duopoly still dominated British broadcast-ing, the relationship between sport and television did begin a gradual process of intensification. In the early 1970s sponsorship, sport and television formed what Whannel (1992) called the sporting triangle, signalling the first steps towards the corporate-media-sport alignment that was to follow. For Boyle and Haynes (2000:44) the 1970s and 1980s were a golden age for British sports television coverage whilst Holt and Mason (1999:120) concluded, 'Spectator sport and the media have fused together. The one is inconceivable without the other'.

However, unlike the US where leagues like the NFL exercised market power, sport in the UK desperately needed television exposure in order to attract sponsorship and boost revenues. In the UK the market for sports broadcasting rights continued to heavily favour the buyers, the broadcasters. In the early 1970s developments in cricket, golf, tennis and Formula 1 illustrated the tensions as sports were being pulled in one direction by out-dated amateur values and organisational structures and, in a new direction, by the increasing influence of market forces and the lure of increased revenues. Ironically, the lack of advertising on the BBC appealed to sponsors and led to a number of sponsored made-for-television cricket events such as John Player Sunday League. British sport began, for the first time, to tentatively embrace commercialism, although the process was usually cautious and gradual (Holt, 1989:354). Profound changes in sport can be linked to a shift in values among the organising elite of sport and the changing role of television, such changes are most apparent in English league football.

English league football rights undervalued

For a long time the staple diet of English league football on television was edited highlights. Between 1968 and 1979 the value of broadcasting rights to football rose to £534,000 a season (Boyle and Haynes, 2004) as the BBC and ITV continued to keep fees depressed. In 1979, ITV tried to break the informal cartel by seeking an exclusive deal for Saturday night football highlights, but the Office of Fair Trading (OFT) intervened and the sought-after slot was subsequently rotated annually between ITV and the BBC. By 1980 broadcasting rights had risen to £2.2 million (Boyle and Haynes, 2004:17), still only a fraction of NFL revenues. With the market still tightly constricted by the ITV–BBC duopoly there was a growing sense among the clubs that English football had undersold itself (Conn, 1997); maybe making more live League football matches available for broadcast would improve revenue streams?

In 1983 Canon became the Football League's first sponsor and the 1983–84 season saw live coverage of League matches return to British television on 2 October 1983 with ITV's *The Big Match Live* – the two-year deal cost £5.2 million for ten matches per season. With the exception of a single match shown on ITV in 1960, remarkably, there had been no live coverage of English league matches prior to this contract, in this respect the UK lagged far behind the US. The 1983 contract is also significant as broadcasters allowed commercial sponsorship for the first time; this took the form of logos displayed on club shirts. With potential revenue from sponsors, and an emerging replica kit market to service, other clubs quickly followed trendsetters Hibernian and Liverpool. By contrast, the NFL has never allowed advertising on team shirts. From today's perspective it is hard to picture English football as unfashionable and out of favour, but it was not the only game in town as athletics provided an unexpected development in British sports broadcasting.

Money matters

In 1984, ITV acquired the rights to broadcast athletics events previously held by the BBC. ITV presented a five-year, £10.5 million deal that was superbly timed as the popular rivalry between middle distance runners Sebastian Coe and Steve Ovett was about to reach its peak. ITV had prized away a key component of BBC Sport's portfolio of rights. The reason for the switch was not criticism of the coverage offered by the BBC, but was the sheer amount of money paid for the broadcasting rights by ITV. With the exception of those events identified on the government's list of protected events, from now on notice was served: whoever could pay the most to acquire broadcasting rights in the UK would win the bidding process.

Back at the Football League in 1985 an offer of £4 million a season for 19 live matches plus highlights was offered jointly by the BBC and ITV. Whilst revenue from television was creeping upwards the game itself was still beset with problems. 1985 provided further crisis points when, between 11 and 29 May, there were tragedies involving loss of life at football stadiums in Bradford City and the Heysel Stadium, Brussels. When, some six months later, the Football League's broadcasting rights deal was finally completed it was for a reduced fee. Significantly, the new contract, which came into effect in 1986, was the first to breach the principle of equal distribution of revenues among all 92-league member clubs (Dobson and Goddard, 2007:81). From now on the rich would get richer.

Live televised league football in the UK

In 1988, the cost of broadcasting rights escalated dramatically when ITV paid £44 million to cover a four-year period from 1989 to 1992; £11 million to show 18 live matches per season. This is a landmark contract in the history of British televised football because, as Boyle and Haynes (2004:19) note, 'it enshrined the notion of live football as an integral part of the regular televisual diet of football supporters'. It was ITV, and not Sky Sports, that raised the number of cameras used for football coverage from around six to 17 per game. In only five years from 1983, the acquisition of broadcasting rights to live coverage of league football had become more sought after than highlights – this is an important shift. And, with challengers to the BBC/ITV duopoly waiting in the wings, the competition to acquire the broadcasting rights to live league football was about to become more intense and more costly than before.

British broadcasting, deregulation and satellite broadcasting

Regulation played a significant part in determining economic practice in media markets and among media firms in the UK. However, competition to the BBC/ITV duopoly, at least as far as sport is concerned, did not come from cable networks but, instead, from direct satellite broadcasting. This was not the supplemental add-on broadcasting model found in the US, it was all or nothing full-on competition for viewers. As Boyle and Haynes (2004) point out, it was not the arrival of ITV in 1955 that signalled the beginning of real commercial competition, but the arrival of BSkyB.

With competition between the BBC and ITV to acquire live football rights already intensifying and an offer of £9 million a season for ten years on the table from BSB (prior to its merger with Sky), the top football clubs were encouraged to form a new super league. According to Conn (1997) club owners reasoned that such a league would increase bargaining power with the broadcasters by creating scarcity; clubs could collect enhanced television revenue and keep these fees for themselves without sharing with teams from the lower divisions. But disaster was to overtake English football again when, in April 1989, 96 fans lost their lives at an FA Cup semi-final match at Hillsborough. The subsequent Taylor Report published in 1990, forced football to rethink its relationship with supporters including the provision of all-seat stadia for top-flight matches. Boyle and Haynes (2000) argue that without the fundamental changes pushed through by the Taylor Report it is doubtful whether commercial television would have shown as much interest in football in the early 1990s as it did.

The FA Premier League

Following the Taylor Report of 1990, Conn takes the view that:

> If football had had a strong governing body, proud, sure of its game and its ethos, to undertake the fullest reassessment of policy called for by Lord Taylor, it would have felt a weighty duty and responsibility to reorganise the game for the good of all who loved it. (Conn, 1997:153)

In the early 1990s, English football was most concerned with economic re-organisation. Even without television revenue unprecedented amounts of money were flooding into the game – Conn (1997) confirms that football was receiving public money in the form of a substantial tax break amounting to £200 million over four years. For Conn, the rush for profit that had become the defining principle of British life in the early 1990s was applied to football by the FA Premier League.

Following a battle for power between the Football League and the Football Association (FA), proposals to unify football from the Football League were rejected and the FA's document *The Blueprint for the Future of Football* (FA, 1991) carried the day. This 118-page document expressed the idea for a breakaway league to serve the richest clubs in England. As such, it set the tone for the takeover of football by businessmen and owners interested in making money from clubs holding assets they viewed as seriously undervalued and from which profit could be realised. For Falcous (2005) the consequences were clear:

> ... these shifts were associated with reconfiguring power relations, the commercial realignment of playing structures, revamped administrative structures and revolutionised spectator provisions and event presentation. The historical legacies of paternalistic amateurism, limited entrepreneurial investment, which had previously constrained commercial activity, and decrepit infrastructures, were rapidly surpassed. (Falcous, 2005:58)

The new league was set up as a corporation owned by the 22-member clubs (20 clubs from 1995 on), each receiving a single vote. The new league also had commercial independence from the Football League and the FA, allowing it to negotiate its own broadcast rights and sponsorship agreements and to route those revenues to the top clubs without sharing with all 92 Football League members. For all the commercial developments driven through by the NFL in the US, it has always retained the principle that clubs shared broadcasting revenue equally.

The FA Premier League was formed on 27 May 1992. Holt and Mason (2000) note the future of football was now in private-hands. Operating as a business, Premier League football now charged what the market could bear to pay for its product and the cost of match tickets rose. On the rehabilitation of football, Dobson and Goddard (2007:69) considered the game's re-emergence: 'the most popular and fashionable national sport was aided by skilful exploitation by the industry of selective aspects of its own heritage'. When considering the creation of the Premier League it should also be noted that this is an extremely rare example of a rival league replacing an incumbent league. The Premier

League overturned the significant advantages held by the dominant league (the Football League); rivals to the NFL in the US have never been so successful.

Premier League broadcasting rights

Recognising that new technology allowed broadcasting rights holders to collect value directly from the consumer – via an encrypted subscription service, lessening the overall reliance on advertising and exploiting the audiences willingness to pay – the BBC saw that it was, effectively, out of the competition to acquire live rights to the Premier League, so it acted strategically by collaborating with BSkyB to offer a joint bid, with the BBC retaining the rights to show match highlights on *Match of The Day*.

Both ITV and BSkyB had lobbied the clubs and the new league intensely in order to secure exclusive live broadcasting rights – Fynn and Guest (1994) and Horsman (1997) provide accounts. ITV's sealed bid was for £262 million. Hearing of this bid from a Premier League official, BSkyB faxed over a revised bid of £304 million for 60 matches per season for five seasons. BSkyB's offer included a top up for overseas rights and a fee for highlights rights provided by the BBC (Horsman, 1997:91–105). This was an increase of £30 million on BSkyB's previous offer, whilst Conn (1997:20) places the BBC contribution as high as £44 million. The previous agreement between the Football League and ITV (1988–92) was £11 million for 18 matches per season, whilst the combined BSkyB/BBC offer for exclusive rights to Premier League matches was an average of £60 million for 60 matches per season, a rise from just over £600,000 per match to around £1 million.

Between 1983 and 1992, the average value of broadcasting rights per match to live League football in England had risen by close to 200%. Top-flight English league football had, some twenty years later than the NFL, come to exercise market power. The UK broadcasting rights market, at least for the Premier League, had become a sellers' market. Economically, live football was more important to the commercial future of BSkyB than it ever was for the BBC. Live Premier League football was scheduled across a range of new kick-off times and was aggressively promoted by Sky Sports. Premier League football was no longer available on free-to-air television in the UK, but was accessed via an annual subscription and additional PPV fees.

The acquisition of sports broadcasting rights, partly due to the remarkable sums now involved, and partly because a number of large transnational corporations dominated the emerging global media markets, was not limited to knowledge of a single market. Gratton and Solberg (2007) suggest that, via News Corporation and FOX, BSkyB was acquainted with the strong competition involved in acquiring sports rights in the US market. This connection may have been influential when BSkyB successfully negotiated a further four-year extension with the Premier League costing £743 million, a 250% rise according to Dobson and Goddard (2007:82). However, it is just as likely to have informed FOX in its acquisition of NFL rights via BSkyB's experience with the Premier League.

The transformation of English league football did not happen in isolation and, among other influences, the rapid growth of global televised sports events, including the IOC Olympics and the FIFA World Cup Finals should be also considered. Of particular significance is the period 1982 to 1986, including the 1984 Los Angeles Olympics (that showcased the growing influence of global corporate interests in televised sport) and the increasing ambition of the organising federations to provide sympathetic television coverage on behalf of their commercial partners.

2.3   The rise of the global televised-sport event

As sports broadcasting developed in the US and UK, economically it was league sport that provided the bread and butter – regular games that were easily scheduled across several months and that delivered predictable audiences for broadcasters. But something new was happening. The shared experience of watching sport on television was becoming an occasion in its own right, particularly with the Olympics and the World Cup Finals broadcast every four years. The IOC Olympic Games and FIFA World Cup Finals grew from modest events to new levels of global prominence primarily through television exposure allied to increasing levels of corporate interest. Four important case studies are now reviewed: the transformation of the IOC Olympic Games (2.3.1), the commercialisation of the FIFA World Cup Finals (2.3.2), the NBA and the global television market (2.3.3) and the UEFA Champions League (2.3.4).

2.3.1   The transformation of the Olympics

The 1968 Mexico Games were the first to attract a significant television audience. For the first time television coverage was in colour and included live slow-motion replays. In the US ABC packaged the games as a dramatic mini-series, a narrative full of human drama and emotion. In the UK, satellite relays enabled the BBC to broadcast breakfast-time

Olympic programmes, a novelty at the time. In 1972, television coverage of the Munich Games was split between sport and news, after eight Palestinian gunmen took eleven Israeli athletes hostage. Despite the tragic death toll, the IOC declared: 'the games must go on'. In 1972, for the first time, the IOC appointed a private advertising agency and sold the rights to use the official Olympic emblem as a marketing tool. However, the Olympic movement nearly collapsed as a consequence of the 1976 Montreal Games. Significantly, the International Olympic Committee (IOC) does not pay to stage the Games. Instead, each Olympics is funded by the host city: a combination of the Local Organising Committee of the Olympic Games and their National Olympic Committee (NOC). Although the event attracted 628 sponsors and suppliers it generated only $7 million for the Local Organising Committee. It took the city 30 years to fully pay off the debt incurred in staging the games, with interest included estimated to be $2 billion (Smit, 2006:184). Hosting an Olympics could be a financial liability.

The Olympics' reputation fell further with the widespread boycott of the 1980 Moscow games. NBC had agreed to pay $87 million for the US television rights before President Carter withdrew the US team in protest over Soviet military action in Afghanistan. The European Broadcasting Union (EBU) obtained rights collectively on behalf of its PSB members so British broadcasters paid much lower rights fees. There was still British television interest in the discredited competition as the British boycott was much less effective than the American one. But the Olympic movement was struggling to find its way. In 1980 Juan Antonio Samaranch was appointed Chairman. Determined to find new sources of revenue, Samaranch proposed to repackage the Olympics to make them more attractive for broadcasters and sponsors. The IOC opted to handle all broadcasting rights negotiations itself, rather than via an agency like International Sport and Leisure (ISL).

According to the IOC, broadcasting rights fees continue to account for 53% of Olympic revenue (IOC, 2009). The majority of this revenue has, since 1980, come from the US free-to-air networks. Revenue from broadcasting rights rose from $287 million in 1984 to $1.706 billion in 2006 – an increase of nearly 600% in 22 years. McCarthy (2014) reports that NBC secured a $7.5 billion deal to broadcast the Olympics between 2021 and 2032, having paid $4.4 billion for the period 2014 to 2020. The turning point for the IOC was the 1984 Los Angeles Games. If the 1980 Moscow Games were an advertisement for state socialism, then the 1984 LA Games were all about the benefits of private enterprise and the neoliberal values of the Reagan-era. The impact of the 1984 Los Angeles

Games on the organisation of sport in general should not be under-estimated. Whilst sponsors had been involved on a small scale since Seiko provided timing support for the 1964 Tokyo Olympics, the age of massive corporate sponsorship of sport had arrived. The US broadcasting rights for the LA Games tripled from $87 million paid by NBC in 1980, to $225 million paid by ABC in 1984. According to Jay (2004) this meant that ABC had to sell more commercials and devote even more airtime to the LA Games in order to recover the broadcasting rights fees and production costs. However, it wasn't the television coverage but the organisation of the Games that was to prove revolutionary.

The Los Angeles committee separated sponsorship into three categories: (a) 34 companies that signed on as Official Sponsors, (b) 64 companies who purchased supplier rights, and (c) 65 companies that were licensees. Each category provided designated rights and exclusivity. The IOC official website confirms that the sponsors were mostly large, multinational corporations – Boyle and Haynes (2000:55) list Coca-Cola, McDonalds, Kodak, Levi-Strauss, Visa and Anheuser-Busch among the official sponsors who paid between $4 million and $15 million each to be associated with the LA Games. More wryly, Jay (2004:181) observes someone even bought the rights to pick up the Olympic garbage. Under its organiser, Peter Ueberroth, over half a billion US dollars was raised and, by making commercial sponsorships such a significant revenue stream, the first-ever privately financed games paid for themselves and turned a profit of $215 million. But this profit did not go to the IOC thus triggering further re-organisation within the Olympic Movement.

By the 1988 Seoul Games the IOC had established its own worldwide marketing programme. The designation worldwide comes from the business categories created for The Olympic Programme (TOP). These are limited to products and services that were considered to be marketable globally. For London 2012 there were 11 TOP worldwide partners (IOC, 2012). Smit (2006) attributes the creation of TOP to the broadcasting rights holding and marketing firm ISL, rather than the IOC. The IOC reasoned that the fewer corporations involved the more valuable individual sponsorships would be. Magdalinski *et al* (2005) note that the IOC benefits as consumers develop brand loyalty to the games, while its TOP partners rely on consumers developing brand loyalty *via* the games. They conclude: 'Perhaps the Olympics *are* more capable of naturalising, even mystifying capitalist relations than are other forms of collective consumption' (Magdalinski *et al*, 2005:52).

Even more so than twenty years of television coverage, what Ueberroth had ultimately achieved with the 1984 Los Angeles games was to reshape the Olympics as a commodity presented to an unprecedented global audience via television. For Jay (2004:182) 'from 1984 the Olympics became a packaged spectacle, an ideal medium through which corporations could sell their products.' And, for Gruneau and Cantelon (1988:347), the change in organisation to a more hierarchical partnership signified the transformation of the Olympics into an increasingly market-orientated project where 'a more fully developed expression of incorporation of sporting practice into the ever-expanding marketplace of international capitalism' is seen. For Boyle and Haynes the step change is significant:

> For many the LA Games were a celebration of corporate capitalism, an arena where human activity was transformed into an economic process that fuelled the consumption of corporate goods and services. It was a process that television both mediated and played a central role in sustaining. Sport had become synonymous with corporate image, television entertainment and consumer capitalism and, for sponsors and marketers, global sporting events would never be the same again. (Boyle and Haynes, 2000:56)

Whilst IOC revenues are now split between the fees they attract for broadcasting rights and a sophisticated marketing plan to promote key sponsors, it is the amalgamation of television and corporate marketing into a *single output* that defines the Olympics. This move was central to the Olympics' transformation over eight years, from a point of near collapse in 1976 to the spectacular growth seen from 1984 on.

2.3.2 The commercialisation of the FIFA World Cup Finals

The governing body for world football, FIFA, was radically transformed between 1974 and 1998. Previously known as an unadventurous organisation, FIFA became a more commercially aligned operation under João Havelange and, as with the Olympics, the 1980s saw significant changes.

From 1982, the FIFA World Cup began to expand. Between 1934 and 1978, 16 national teams took part in the World Cup Finals (and 15 in 1938) before the competition was expanded to 24 teams in 1982 and 32 teams in 1998. The FIFA World Cup was first televised in 1954 and the primary sale of broadcasting rights was to the World TV consortium of public broadcasters with the European Broadcasting Union (EBU) leading the negotiations (Jennings, 2006). This arrangement remained unchallenged until 1996 when FIFA, advised by ISL, was convinced that the PSB monopoly led by the EBU was acquiring broadcasting rights for well under the potential market value – without demand created by competition, prices for broadcasting rights remained relatively deflated. Unlike the Olympics, there was virtually no demand from US broadcasters for the World Cup. On the other hand, the massive audiences attracted to the free-to-air terrestrial PSBs had tremendous appeal to potential corporate sponsors. Paradoxically, achieving the highest price for broadcasting rights did not necessarily deliver the most profitable outcome to FIFA.

FIFA's transformation was initially linked to the rapid expansion of the football marketing business, but it is the subsequent amalgamation of: (a) the interests of large corporate sponsors with, (b) sympathetic event management and television coverage that (c) provides access to mass audiences that is significant. FIFA's own sales pitch says: 'Together with the official broadcasters who deliver worldwide TV and radio coverage of the events, the sponsors and licensees are the pillars that support the staging and promotion of a FIFA event' (FIFA, 2009).

During the 1970s and 1980s the football marketing business was largely formed by two men: Patrick Nally and Horst Dassler, son of Adi Dassler the founder of the Adidas sporting goods firm. Nally advised sports organisers how to package their events in ways that would be appealing to broadcasters and sponsors then he would persuade companies like Coca-Cola to become sponsors of these events. Ahead of the 1982 World Cup, Nally set out a formal sponsorship practice titled *Intersoccer* that identified exactly what rights would be accorded to sponsors and how these rights would be protected on their behalf (Nally, 1979). *Intersoccer* was broadly similar to Ueberroth's three-tier structure for the 1984 LA Olympics; it became a widely influential template.

Nally also cooperated with Dassler at the 1978 World Cup in Argentina selling advertising space, but Dassler became convinced it was the business of sports broadcasting rights that had the greatest potential (Smit, 2006). Up to this point, no third party company beyond a sports federation or broadcasters had held the broadcasting rights to a major sports event. Dassler jettisoned Nally and teamed up with the Japanese advertising giant Dentsu. In the autumn of 1982, a marketing and broadcasting rights holding company called International Sport and Leisure (ISL) was set up in Lucerne, Switzerland and jointly owned by Dassler and Dentsu (Smit, 2006). The new firm quickly corralled the football marketing business.

Anecdotally it is said that Dassler taught Havelange how to sell the World Cup and Samaranch how to market the Olympics. Dassler continued to advise Havelange and, from 1982, FIFA greatly expanded its commercial ventures, including advertising and merchandising. ISL paid 45 million Swiss francs for the 1986 World Cup in Mexico and they raised over 200 million Swiss francs from assorted sponsors, profit that went directly to FIFA, unlike the relationship between Los Angeles 1984 and the IOC (Smit, 2006:196). In 1988, the award of the 1994 World Cup to the US appeared to underline FIFA's interest in profit and engaging corporate interests.

According to Smit, for several years ISL were issued huge broadcasting rights contracts for both the Olympics and the World Cup Finals without a second thought given to the process (Smit, 2006:196). For the first time, broadcasting rights from sports governing bodies were held by a third party for subsequent sale to broadcasters without the need for ISL to make any programmes – it can be argued that the creation of value, as a separate process from production, reflected the general swing away from the production of goods to the provision of services that was taking place in the wider economy. The ISL operation was a trailblazer for other rights holding companies, including IMG, Kirch Media and SportFive.

As was the case with the Olympics, the World Cup Finals were redefined in ways that mostly benefited FIFA. This included placing the marketing strategies of large transnational corporations at the very heart of tournament staging and television presentation. In a set up reminiscent of The Olympic Programme (TOP) signing a group of primary sponsors was designed to (a) spread the financial risk of the World Cup Finals, and (b) result in less dependence on revenue from the sale of broadcasting rights alone. However, the two activities remain intricately linked. The conversion of the governing institution of football into a corporate organisation that, for example, now hedges against variations in currency exchange valuations, or that requests tax-free status and fast-track work permits when operating in a host country (Jennings, 2006) is part of the overall transformation. (The reiteration of claims made by Jennings in a Panorama documentary titled 'FIFA's Dirty Secrets' shown on BBC One on 29 November 2010 was controversial at the time but appears vindicated by the involvement of the FBI in 2015).

The ISL–FIFA joint marketing strategy provided a commercial base from which international football, now being sold as a highly commercialised entertainment industry and marketed as 'the World's game', could extend its relationship with the transnational corporate world. In other words, the four-year period between 1982 and 1986 saw a new corporate–sport–media axis emerge that enabled the dramatic rise of global televised sport events from the mid-1980s well into the twenty-first century. As the rest of the sports world assimilated these new business models, the next step was their adoption by national and regional sports federations.

2.3.3   The NBA, sports marketing and globalisation

The NBA was the first league to align their television product with growing global marketing trends. Entertainment values and an overt association between celebrity and sports superstars were key ingredients in the NBA brand.

In the early 1980s, the NBA came very close to collapse (Jay, 2004:202). The increase in competition, particularly from new media providers, to acquire sports broadcasting rights was critical to the NBA's development and came at a very opportune time. In 1984, David Stern, a practising lawyer, was appointed NBA Commissioner. Four months later Michael Jordan was drafted into the NBA by the Chicago Bulls. Jordan's rise to global superstardom is attributed to David Falk, also a lawyer, and the ProServ agency. ProServ set up Jordan Universal Marketing and Promotions (JUMP) wrapping Jordan's commercial activities into a corporation. Jordan's popularity was enhanced through his endorsement of Nike sports products. Falk persuaded Nike to create a signature shoe for Jordan called 'Air Jordan' (Jay, 2004). From 1985, Air Jordan shoes were advertised widely on television. The commercials shot by movie director Spike Lee, who appeared in the commercials reiterating his Mars Blackmon character from the 1986 movie *She's Gotta Have It*, achieved cult status and were instrumental in propelling the increasingly commercial culture of modern sport into the mainstream. Jordan's example illustrates how athletic ability was no longer enough to define top sports stars; 'they also needed to promote themselves, to turn their skills into something that sells' (Jay, 2004:241). By 1992 only $4 million came from the Chicago Bulls, with another $21 million from McDonalds, Coca-Cola, Wheaties, Haynes and Gatorade.

Off the back of Jordan's success the NBA adopted an aggressive global marketing strategy. Nike founder Phil Knight suspected that the NBA was free-riding on the advertising campaigns of Nike as the league set about constructing its own personality-based sports brand. In selling NBA broadcasting rights abroad, the NBA had an advantage over the NFL insofar as basketball was played more widely elsewhere than American football. *NBA Entertainment* also produced a number of in-house basketball magazine and lifestyle programmes. *NBA Inside Stuff* was one of several well-produced programmes supported by substantial budgets that were offered as a bundle to international broadcasters, often for free (subject to a guarantee of a reasonably prominent slot in the schedules) when rights to live coverage of regular NBA games were purchased. The extra programmes added value to the rights packages and helped spread the NBA message. 'That's the beauty of television', explained Stern (Jay, 2004:229). 'Other brands have to buy their way on through advertising. Our core product is a two-hour commercial that someone pays us to run.' For Stern, then, NBA games were used to drive the NBA's global commercial activities. As part of the marketing process dozens of A-list Hollywood stars plugged the league by repeating the NBA's marketing mantra 'I love this game' to camera whilst watching the action from expensive courtside seats. Stars like Bill Murray (Chicago), Jack Nicholson (LA Lakers) and Spike Lee (NY Knicks) were frequently picked out during live coverage as ideas about sports, entertainment, celebrity, superstardom and commercialism began to merge.

The epitome of the personality-basketball-sporting goods marketing formula came in 1992 with the appearance of the NBA Dream Team at the Barcelona Olympics. Twelve of the highest paid professional basketball players were selected as national pride and commercial goals became fused together. The Dream Team won gold spurring the NBA's global commercial activities on to a peak in the mid-1990s. Initially a US domestic league, the NBA worked hard to create a global market for sports broadcasting rights that extended beyond quadrennial events like the Olympics and World Cup. Executives of the newly formed Premier League were attentive to the NBA's commercial activities in the mid-1990s. The Premier League's chief executive, Rick Parry, reviewed NBA operations at its base in Secaucus, NJ. Parry was accompanied by representatives from Chrysalis Sport (an independent production company) where I was producer of NBA coverage for Channel Four.

2.3.4 UEFA Champions League, embedded sponsorship and output control

UEFA is one of the six regional federations within FIFA, it runs a number of high-profile football competitions at national and at club level. In 1955, the newly formed UEFA came up with a bold formula for football that combined, (a) mid-week football matches held under new floodlighting systems, (b) improving airline services to transport clubs to matches across Europe, and (c) emerging pan-European television coverage.

By the early 1990s Europe's leading clubs were threatening to form their own European super league. In response UEFA introduced a league system that guaranteed all qualifying clubs a minimum number of games, with these games came additional revenue. A dedicated company – The Event Agency and Marketing AG (TEAM Marketing) – was formed in 1991 to secure 'the greatest monetary gain through marketing of television rights and sponsorship opportunities of the UEFA Champion's League' (Sugden and Tomlinson, 1998:93–97). The approach adopted by UEFA and TEAM Marketing owed much to the models created for the 1984 Los Angeles Olympics, Nally's influential *InterSoccer* template and by the activities of FIFA and ISL. The new Champions League format was launched in the 1992–93 season. By 1998, TEAM Marketing was estimated to receive £30 million from the competition per year, from an estimated income of £185 million to UEFA with the participating clubs sharing £100 million (Banks, 2002:128).

What distinguishes the UEFA Champions League is that television coverage comes with an onscreen presence for UEFA's 'official' corporate sponsors (8 in 2014–15) already attached. Guaranteed exposure for UEFA's commercial partners is embedded within a highly prescribed television production and event-wide presentation methodology. Acquiring the broadcasting rights to the Champions League means that broadcasters must follow the procedures and practices set out in the UEFA Champions League Production Manual. The manual has grown to nearly 150 pages (2013–2014 season); it is written by TEAM Marketing and describes all aspects of Matchday (-1) and Matchday television coverage and distribution in detail. It also includes timed multi-lateral running orders that all broadcasters must follow pre-match, in and out of each half, at half-time and at full-time. TEAM Marketing executives are present at every match to advise the host broadcaster; they also monitor the television coverage for every Champions League match. The UEFA Champions League host broadcast operation represents an unprecedented level of control exerted by a governing body over the broadcast output on behalf of its corporate sponsors. 'Developments in the commercial and media world have gone hand in hand with football's evolution in recent years. Consequently, UEFA's marketing, commercial and technological activities have intensified considerably' (UEFA, 2009). Alex Fynn, one of the original architects of the Premier League (Boyle and Haynes, 2004:64), claims UEFA 'Now recognise through control of sponsorship, advertising and TV rights, that they have the power'. Such market power goes a very long way to define what sports we can see, where we can see them and what the final programmes look and sound like.

Conclusion

This chapter argued that sport and television in the UK have become realigned along commercial and consumer-oriented structures more typically seen in the US. This is despite starting from virtually opposite positions post-World War II. The Premier League now demonstrates unprecedented levels of corporate organisation and profit-driven motivation, surpassing some of the activities of the NFL, a League that has set the benchmark for commercial activity.

The comparison between the development of sport and television in the US and UK addresses a surprising gap in understanding and that underlines the scale and the speed with which sport and television in the UK has changed. It also embraces the 'peculiar economics of sport' (Neale, 1964) a critical dimension frequently overlooked in political economy interpretations.

From 1945 until 1970 British sport was pulled between an idealised amateur past and a commercialised free-market future – a legacy is found in the British government's list of protected sports events. However, from 1970 the development of sport in the UK was increasingly influenced by the combined needs of television, sponsorship and advertising. In the late 1980s significant technological and regulatory change subjected sport and broadcasting in the UK to free market principles.

It was argued that the behaviour of the NFL was very significant. The 1964 Tokyo Olympics are commonly held to have triggered an escalation in rights fees, but a more convincing argument arises from the consequences of competition between the three major US networks to acquire NFL broadcasting rights. The NFL was the first professional sports league to understand the importance of (a) the collective sale of sports broadcasting rights (cartel behaviour), (b) providing league-wide sporting equilibrium (competitive balance and uncertainty of outcome), and (c) exercising its market power to collect this value. As there was no effective substitute for the NFL it became a seller's market and the price of NFL rights rose steadily from the 1970s. Economists including Fort (2006) have identified the willingness to pay of sponsors and advertisers to access audiences as highly significant in (a) determining what content is broadcast, and (b) in changing the revenue side of sports forever.

It was also argued that the NBA, in the 1980s, overtly allied its sport product to entertainment values and celebrity endorsements that, together, helped to propel the commercial culture of modern sport into the mainstream.

The 1980s also saw the formalisation of large-scale corporate sponsorship as a viable alternative to advertising. This had a profound impact on the growth of global televised sports events including the Olympics and the World Cup Finals. From a point of near collapse, the IOC set out to make the Olympic Games more appealing to broadcasters and large corporate sponsors. The amalgamation of sport, television and corporate interests into a *single package* was commercially successful and, from the landmark 1984 Los Angeles Games, the IOC moved forward on a more aggressively commercial basis. Similarly, FIFA greatly increased its revenues from advertising, sponsorship and broadcasting rights from the early 1980s, with the biggest gains coming from 1986 onwards. International Sport and Leisure (ISL) was an influential company in developing lucrative methods of sports marketing for the IOC and FIFA. The company also pioneered the third party acquisition of sports broadcasting rights and how to sell these rights on to media providers. In 1992, the UEFA Champions League was launched as it adopted many of the lessons learned by the IOC and FIFA. UEFA required participating broadcasters to follow their highly prescribed Production Manual and to ensure that the embedded sponsorship from UEFA's key commercial partners was correctly woven into the coverage.

In the UK, the BBC/ITV broadcasting duopoly operating in tandem with the government's list of protected events had stifled the value of sports rights, with live football remaining undervalued until the late 1980s. However, as was the case in the US over a decade earlier, a combination of technological development and deregulation rapidly changed the broadcasting landscape. In the UK this meant the 1990 Broadcasting Act and the arrival of direct satellite broadcasting. BSkyB did not see itself as *supplemental* to the existing broadcaster order but sought to overturn the established players and dominate the market – an era of fierce commercial competition had begun. In 1992 the creation of the Premier League signalled the most rational approach to capital accumulation yet by a British sport. With its corporate structure and commercial autonomy the Premier League is driven by an unambiguous profit motive. In some important ways it can be argued that the Premier League has become even more commercial and profit-driven than the NFL, both in terms of its structure where members act as shareholders and the global sales revenues for broadcasting rights it has achieved.

The undertow is how economic, political and technological forces combined in various ways from the early 1970s to create a world where what is good for business is considered to be good for us all. 'Neoliberalism ...' claimed Harvey (2005:166), '... has unquestionably rolled back the bounds of commodification and greatly extended the reach of legal contracts'. Among the consequences was the 'financialisation of everything' (2005:33). By the early 1990s, sport had come to matter a great deal to big business and managers of increasingly commercial and global media industries. 'Sports now stress the need to be business-like and efficient, offer sites for the celebration of corporate capitalism ... and, in general have become prime sites for the construction and reproduction of an entrepreneurial culture', concludes Whannel (1992:208). For professional sport this meant realignment with the interests of corporate investment and the managerial tenets of advertising, marketing and public relations (Falcous, 2005).

The US market structure has meant that the Major League sports have retained a strong presence on the free-to-air broadcast networks. The model of increased exposure and higher audience ratings via free-to-air television has served the interests of teams, leagues, broadcasters, advertisers, sponsors and viewers alike. It is ironic that free-to-air broadcasting provided the foundations on which the highly commercialised modern sports industry is built to the extent, today, that media regulation, in the form of listed events protection, and competition law is all that has prevented wholesale migration to pay-TV in the UK.

This chapter provided important background context prior to the discussion of technology, broadcasting rights and regulation that follows.

3
Technology

How three largely unseen upstream pre-production processes increasingly shape television sport is examined with dedicated chapters that consider technology, broadcasting rights (including the economics of sports organisations and media providers) and regulation (politics). The sheer scale of transformations since the late 1980s is illustrated, including how a significant increase in demand has been met by a combination of digital technology and new production methods.

Throughout the history of television sport, technology has played a pivotal role; with the exception of news production, no other television genre is so closely associated with technological developments and logistical aspects of coverage than sport. Evens, Iosifidis and Smith (2013) identify three phases in the history of television in the UK: 1) public service regulated monopoly/duopoly (under conditions of spectrum scarcity), 2) from the 1980s to the mid-1990s the emergence of new delivery systems, the end of public service duopoly and the introduction of commercial competition and, 3) the current phase, the transition from analogue to digital. As technological developments embrace (a) transmission, including new viewing options, (b) production, (c) distribution, and (d) archive, the position adopted here is not in favour of technological determinism but for viewing transformation as part of a wider process of marketisation and how the market has become the central frame of reference for cultural activity (Boyle and Haynes, 2004:52).

Examining broadcasting we can see: (a) the platforms, technology and workflows used for transmission, and (b) the services that are presented on these platforms: the schedules and content. Increased demand for sports content comes from broadcasters and pay-TV providers, who are not broadcasters in the traditional sense. Looking at production technology, whilst this may initially be considered a third category of activity, recent convergence – particularly the widespread adoption of digital media servers – means the boundaries between transmission, production and distribution have narrowed substantially.

This chapter considers the current phase, the transformation from analogue to digital HD and, crucially, how digital technology became the basis for new methods of production, including how accelerated workflows deliver dramatic increases in the volume and scope of content in television sport. As most political economy discussion tends to focus on the demand side – on the creation and ownership of content and channels – a supply side perspective is provided here; of how radical developments in sports production technology were essential in meeting a rapidly escalating demand for sports content. Meeting this demand would not have been possible working in the analogue paradigm. Also of interest is *who* is using new technology, *how* it is used and for what purposes, *why*. The extent to which football, and the Premier League in particular, has entered a new phase of intense commodification is remarkable and is illustrated in a case study. As Doyle (2002) notes, the continuous expansion in the ways in which television can be distributed to viewers is significant. The ways very large volumes of content is (a) received by broadcasters, (b) organised into recognisable schedules, and (c) disseminated in a structured way is now reviewed.

3.1 Transmission technology

It was the creation of viable alternatives to previously limited and strictly controlled analogue frequencies that radically changed television broadcasting in the UK. The volume of available sports content, plus the numerous ways this content can be consumed has been transformed in 20 years, with a great deal of momentum added in the past decade. Such processes, argues Schimmel (2005:3), accelerate 'the commodification and commercialisation of sport and deliver sport product on ever increasing scales to international consumers'. A vanguard of technological change was transmission operations.

1992, analogue, tape-based transmission systems

By the early 1990s terrestrial broadcasters had developed well-understood transmission processes that did not vary much. This was an analogue, tape-based operation where workflows were determined by the hardware that was used to organise and transmit content. Broadcasters acquired content on videotape. Tapes were barcoded, given a quality control check and copied for transmission. Presentation schedules contained interstitials, channel-branding, content promotion, information and programme links. Commercial broadcasters incorporated advertisements into their schedules. With robotic machines (Odetics) or flexicarts physically moving media into place it was a straightforward mechanical operation. In transmission, physical tapes and play-out machines were visible assets and content could be seen as it progressed through linear workflow towards a live broadcast output controlled via a dedicated transmission area and supervised by a presentation director or transmission controller. For example, each BBC channel had a dedicated transmission suite with an on-air presentation director, production assistant and technical staff. However, computer software and new digital, server-based technology would soon trigger the re-organisation and eventual automation of transmission systems.

Beyond traditional terrestrial TV

From 1993, the established terrestrial broadcasting order in the UK faced a number of challenges with new channels launching and innovative ways of consuming content becoming available. On 1 September 1993, the BSkyB multi-channel satellite service was launched. BSkyB introduced monthly subscriptions and the electronic turnstile or pay-per-view broadcasting. By 1996 660,000 customers each paid a one-off fee to watch a boxing match between Frank Bruno and Mike Tyson. But this was still an analogue service; it ran until September 2001 when it was superseded by the Sky Digital platform.

All broadcasting systems are essentially downlink transmissions. Linear broadcasters offer programmes in a fixed schedule, a timed sequence used to order content. But ideas about viewing content were starting to change, options surrounding choice of content and about when this content could be viewed, were becoming available. Notable steps include:

- In 1994, the arrival of Amazon, 1995 saw DVD and in 1997 the TiVo personal hard disk recorder arrived.
- In October 1998 BSkyB launched an all-digital satellite service, including an interactive red-button service now known as Sky Active.
- In 2001 the Sky+ box was launched.
- With the new millennium came Google, the iPod and Xbox. 2002 saw the launch of RIM's Blackberry popular email-linking service. Internet 2.0 helped establish iTunes (April 2003), Facebook, Flickr and Gmail all of which followed in 2004.

- In 2005, Sky News and Sky Sports were streamed to mobile phones. The first YouTube video was uploaded in April 2005. Videos and TV shows were available to download at the iTunes store.
- In 2006, Sky+ HD became the UK's first nationwide high-definition service. The online social networking and micro blogging service, Twitter, was launched.
- 2008 saw the BBC and ITV offer a joint-venture service on Freesat, a UK oriented free-to-air digital satellite service.
- From 2010, BSkyB offered a 3-D service, the BBC followed but both were short lived due to lack of demand.

Turning to mobile platforms, a significant incentive to advertisers using Internet and mobile services was the ability to collect more detailed data, including customer usage and preferences. The iPhone was launched in 2007. In 2010 Apple launched the iPad, this type of device is attributed with establishing a notable change in viewing habits as more media, including television content, could now be accessed wirelessly.

A range of video on demand (VOD) services were also introduced. The BBC iPlayer had been around since 2005, going live on 25 December 2007, and Sky Anytime+ was launched in 2010. By 2011, the BBC iPlayer included links to programmes from other broadcasters – the ITV Player, 4oD and Demand 5. Specific iPlayer applications for mobile platforms were launched in February 2011. Sky Go, also launched in 2011, enabled its customers to watch live television on the move via laptops, smartphones and tablets as part of their monthly subscription.

During this period the value of live sport, particularly football continued to rise – for media providers there was no viable substitute. 2012 saw BT Sport enter the market for sports rights – BT's intention was to use high profile sports content to drive customers towards using its fibre-based services. The old analogue system was switched off in 2012 and by 2013 content could now be viewed via:

- Digital satellite television
- Cable television
- Digital terrestrial television
- IPTV
- Laptop, mobile and tablet
- DVD

A range of enhanced television broadcasting developments had also been introduced, including:

- TV anytime, viewer-determined consumption utilising time shifting
- TV anywhere, content viewed via laptop and tablet computers, plus smart phones
- Interactivity, viewers could participate by giving comments, voting and receiving additional information on VOD programmes. Smart TVs were Internet compatible, connecting via the TV receiver, set-top-box, broadband router or a manufacturer application.

Against a backdrop of wider change, the ways broadcasters organised and transmitted their content began to move on from established and largely manual methods.

The transition to digital transmission

From the mid-1990s broadcasters began to introduce software and digital media server-based systems to control key aspects of the transmission workflow. A broadcast technology expert, speaking in 2013, confirmed these media servers 'enabled true multi-channel broadcasting, which was never possible using videotape'. It is the ability to *simultaneously* broadcast several channels to different territories that is significant, particularly for multinational broadcasters including Discovery Networks. Early in the new millennium media servers became pivotal to transmission operations. As more affordable media storage and more powerful servers became available, managers realised that more media could be placed on the central server for play out; a senior transmission manager recalls how servers were introduced:

> Although tape formats remained for long form programme material and for interstitials, by 2000 or so, commercials in the UK were being delivered on MPEG2 files to play out providers. These files required boxes to receive material and servers to store the high-resolution files. (Senior broadcast transmission manager, 2013)

By using specialist scheduling software, transmission could be fully automated. In 2002 Quantel introduced scalable hardware and software solutions that combined browsing and broadcasting at the same time – again, when working with large volumes of content, it is the ability to do different things at the same time that is significant.

In 2004, the first ingest-to-air workflow automation was introduced and, from 2005, broadcasters began to ingest their entire broadcast content onto central servers. But transmission was not yet tapeless; the reliability of Digital Betacam systems moderated the introduction of file-based systems, plus broadcasters' libraries were still full of videotape. Tapes were used for making copies of programmes and for re-versioning purposes, including providing different language versions or versions with subtitles. Unlike tapes, which were visible assets, file-based content had to be ingested with the correct metadata attached otherwise it could disappear on the system. Speaking in 2013, a director of transmission notes: 'storing and transferring files, particularly via the Internet, also raised the risk of piracy'; this remains a global concern among media providers.

The digital hangover

The transition from analogue to digital transmission has been beset with operational issues. These can involve *codecs*, the structure used to create a file; *transcoding*, or the transfer of a file from one format to another, and *encoding*, the creation of a file when content has been transferred from videotape. As different files are created using different codecs, difficulties in reading files can arise; transmission experts confirm incompatibility was a wide-ranging problem in transmission suites at all media providers. Media Asset Management (MAM) systems were introduced to help move files through the full transmission workflow, from receipt and ingesting, quality control, encoding and transcoding, playout, repurposing and archiving. However, speaking in 2014, an experienced Director of Transmission had 'yet to see a system that offers a definitive benchmark in reliability and performance'. An unwanted by-product in the proliferation of content delivery platforms is a loss of a common operational standard across the array of file-based formats now used, in other words the more platforms using file-based media there are, the more confusion is created.

Digital expansion

Digital transmission saw the number of channels available in the UK increase dramatically. In 1992 there had been four terrestrial broadcast channels; 22 years later the Sky platform alone listed 36 exclusively sports-based channels. BSkyB and BT are engaged in communications technology convergence. BSkyB offers television, broadband, Wi-Fi and telephone services, as does BT; both use high profile sports content to attract customers. All major terrestrial broadcasters offer additional viewing platforms like iPlayer for viewing content, either live or on demand. And beyond that, providers like Yahoo offer clip-based content services, many of which can be viewed streamed on national newspaper sites.

From this brief overview we can take away the following points:

1) The tapeless transmission workflows adopted by many broadcasters do not offer a fully coherent path from content creation through to final broadcast.
2) Quality levels for different outputs has expanded, making it impractical for all output to be delivered from a single point. Workflows must take into account the various ways that content is to be used, as this varies significantly from platform to platform.
3) There has been a rise in multinational broadcasters that simultaneously provide global markets with repurposed content, from very large providers like Discovery Networks and NBC Universal to microbroadcasters like Paris-based Trace Sports. As many as 13 versions may need to be derived from the original to service different markets.
4) The ability of domestic UK media providers to handle many more feeds has allowed additional pop-up channels, or where, for example, Sky Sports viewers, in the 2014–15 season, could choose to watch up to 8 UEFA Champions League matches at the same time via the red button option.

These developments are relevant because (a) transmission was the first area to adopt digital server technology, (b) sport is an important driver in the take up of new broadcasting technology, (c) live sport broadcasting rights have escalated in value due to increased demand, (d) the distribution of television content has generally become much more specialised, (e) content can be more tightly focussed on smaller groups of consumers, particularly via pay-TV, and (f) further consumption data can be tracked and compiled and this, in itself, has a financial value to broadcasters as they sell access to audiences, to sponsors and advertisers.

3.2   Production technology, the analogue paradigm

In the early 1990s sports production workflows were constrained within an analogue paradigm, this section explains the limits of analogue technology and production methods including an indicative workflow from 1992. This football production workflow is used to benchmark the transformation from analogue to digital and to pinpoint how production methods have changed.

Analogue technology and tape-based workflows

The key limitations of analogue technology and workflows are particularly evident when looking at videotape recording, videotape editing, graphics inputs and audio recording.

In 1992 videotape was the primary medium on which to record, edit, play out and archive sports content. Incremental advances were made, like variable replay speeds and increased portability of smaller formats (like Sony Betacam) and videotape operations remained at the heart of all sports productions and was often referred to as the 'engine room'. The two most obvious limitations of analogue videotape are 1) the ability to make copies (this was done in real time and introduced deterioration with each copy made), and in 2) editing, where the fixed timelines of videotape were very restrictive. Once an edit was made the timeline was fixed, it wasn't possible to replace one sequence with a longer or shorter sequence as it was with film, where the edited sequence is literally cut open and the new sequence inserted. As sports content was mostly prepared using 2 machines, then creating a wipe or a mix, rather than a cut, was troublesome and involved copying material to a third machine. An independent production company, Cheerleader Productions, introduced three-machine video editing to sport; three-machine editing was more typically found in entertainment programmes and US sports presentations.

Videotape recordings were crucially important and a hand-written log sheet accompanied each tape. This was a description of all content 'logged' along the timeline (typically time-of-day timecode that looks like a digital clock), the log was made by an assistant producer during recording and was the only method of knowing what was on each tape, if the log was lost the tape was useless until re-logged.

For graphics, input was mostly limited to the Aston caption generator, with the Chyron equivalent providing a bolder US style. The telestrator was an infrequently used device that allowed a commentator to draw basic lines on screen (i.e., over a video replay) to highlight relevant action. As this was used on US television it was not encouraged in the UK. However, BBC Sport became an early-adopter of digital technology when it introduced a computer-based results service in the late 1980s. The system was able to handle very quick data input – for example Saturday afternoon football results (when most games were still played on a Saturday afternoon) – and tie this input (the scores) to pre-designed fixtures lists allowing for much quicker presentation to air.

Finally, audio recording and mixing was subject to the same generic limitations as videotape editing. Recording was restricted to the number of tracks available on videotape. As new tape formats like Betacam were introduced, even recording basic stereo became challenging (due to limited tracks) so, in some important respects, audio recording was very limited for a while. However, in 1993, audio provided an introduction to digital technology for many producers. The ability of digital audio mixing to move material around on the timeline felt revolutionary in the flexibility it offered.

Experienced producers recall that, in most respects, working in analogue demanded conscious preparation (finding tapes, logs and timecodes) and was generally laborious and slow to achieve even modest results.

Typical workflows, 1992

Turning to football for an example of the analogue paradigm, around six cameras were typically used on any match. Of these, at least two would have long telephoto lenses to provide close ups of players and reactions of managers (figure 3.1).

For a six camera outside broadcast, using three videotape replay machines was typical. Any videotape replays required the machine to stop recording, spool back and re-cue the action before it was ready to play back at a reduced speed. The mixer console handled camera and graphics inputs and offered a variety of transitions from cuts to wipes. A typical desk would have a maximum of 48 inputs and a single graphics source. A separate, smaller truck would be on location to handle onwards distribution of output, via BT Tower to the broadcaster's base.

An outside broadcast of this nature could be self-contained and would not require a large number of production staff; normally a producer (or producer/director), an assistant producer and a production assistant would suffice. For the BBC, outside broadcasts were not often standalone, but part of a larger presentation, such as *Grandstand* or *Match of The Day*, but even the BBC's flagship football magazine was not an onerously complex production.

Match of The Day (MoTD) was presented from a dedicated sports studio at Television Centre. A programme editor ran the production with an assistant editor, a studio producer/director, production assistant and a team of assistant producers in the videotape area preparing match action and any analysis clips for broadcast.

Key to the MoTD operation was a network of incoming lines that carried feeds of each game back to Television Centre. From 1992 this included shared feeds from games covered by Sky Sports, but minus Sky's

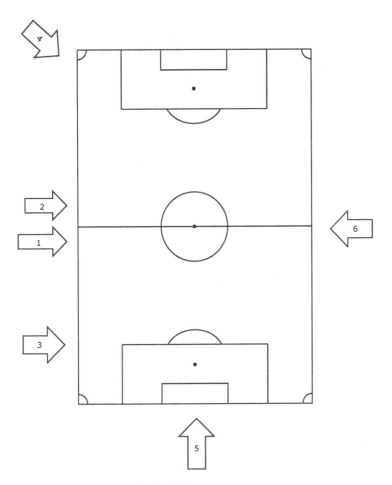

Figure 3.1 Six camera plan for football

commentary team, graphics and video effects – known as a clean feed. As each game was received an assistant producer would log the action, using timecode as a reference, then work with a VT editor to edit the match to duration.

Match of the Day typically broadcast three matches, and, from 1992, included a roundup of the goals scored at all other matches. Each segment was routed to the studio via the VT multiplexer, a switching device that handled a large number of VT inputs, but offered just two outputs to the studio gallery. A senior assistant producer, or for bigger productions a VT producer, would run the multiplexer to ensure the correct content reached the studio. After each broadcast, tapes and log sheets were gathered for archiving the key recordings in the sports library.

A bit like the practices previously used in transmission, equipment behaved as expected and worked well (within its limits) and these methods were seldom subject to much in the way of change.

Live Premier League football, Sky Sports style

In 1988 ITV acquired the rights to show 18 live league matches a year. Coverage escalated from six cameras to 17. As a result Boyle and Haynes (2004:19) consider ITV to have raised the status of live football coverage, but it was the launch of the Premier League on Sky Sports that really moved the goalposts. From August 1992 Sky Sports offered live and exclusive coverage of 60 live Premier League matches per year. In terms of technology, a significant change was the introduction of subscription-based broadcasting that used encryption of the satellite signal as a turnstile to allow viewers access. Reviewing production technology, the Sky Sports formula was less about new technology than using *more* of the existing technology and doing so in different ways.

Several aspects of coverage immediately stood out: the introduction of the game clock and the always on score caption, a consistently high number of cameras covering action, more close ups including the use of Steadicam harness system along the touchline, the prominent Quantel swoop (with sound effects) that accompanied replays, more frequent use of reverse angle replays, and Sky Sport's distinctive graphics. But the presentation style was not entirely new, as a dedicated sports channel executive observes:

> Sky went about copying a variety of styles and looks from US TV and rolled them out in the UK, including presenters looking to camera and presenting styles that were direct lifts from US TV. (Sports channel executive, 2012)

The similarities with US sports broadcasting did not end there, some programme titles even sounded American, including *The Monday Night Football* taken from ABC's long-running NFL flagship *Monday Night Football*, or *Super Sunday* again used on NFL. In 1993 US broadcaster ESPN was seriously considering legal action against Sky's *Sports Centre* for alleged format copyright infringement. Where Sky Sports did begin a new chapter in television coverage was with more detailed match analysis, in part this was due to the additional time the channel had to fill. Also evident was an aggressive new marketing philosophy used to promote the Sky Sports brand.

For Sky Sports it was the *different* ways technology was used that is more significant than what was used. In ways that are reminiscent of ABC executive Roone Arledge's up close and personal philosophy, Sky Sports used more technology as it sought to stand out. Soon competing channels were promoting key points of difference in their coverage to lure potential customers. Speaking in an article in the Daily Telegraph (18 April 2011) Andy Melvin, then Sky Sports deputy-managing director, captured the mood:

> I had spent 10 years covering football in Glasgow where everyone looked down on sports broadcasting as an irrelevance. TV then was dominated by luvvies and by news junkies, neither of whom had the slightest interest in sport. But then I joined Sky and felt we had been given this incredible opportunity.
>
> It was a huge gamble, and the sceptics said, 'This will be shit TV, real lowbrow stuff'. But we were a team of football people, making programmes for football people, and we were determined to make it work. (Briggs, 2011)

The mantra was more, but just how far could outside broadcast operations grow? As an independent producer I recall how outside broadcast trucks began to literally expand sideways to accommodate more equipment and people. At the biggest sports events there were separate trucks for the gallery, another housing videotape operations, sometimes yet another truck to control the presentation studio output. In terms of videotape operations, it was possible to increase the number of inputs but that meant increasing the number of tape machines and finding (a) a place to put them, (b) means of wiring them into the system, and (c) managing the mountains of tape recordings generated. The analogue paradigm soon presented a very real physical limit to what could be achieved. The sheer size of equipment racks, the amount of cabling, the number of logging and editing stations, the ability to input raw material from different sources, including more and more cameras, into more powerful mixing desks, plus the ability to output the final programme could only expand so far.

Vertical integration or free market provision of technology?

A change in the impetus in the development of production technology in the UK can also be noted in the 1990s. Historically, technical support for studios, outside broadcasts and editing systems was a matter of vertical integration, particularly at the BBC where virtually all aspects of technology, engineering and logistics were all under one roof – or at least one metaphorical roof. To some extent the regional ITV companies replicated this as they shared resources. Whilst BSkyB had built their own matrix of incoming and outgoing lines, editing and studio facilities at their base in Isleworth, significantly the company did not invest in outside broadcast equipment and, instead, chose to rely on external firms to provide technology for location use. This clearly reduced the need for large-scale capital investment whilst allowing access to the newest equipment as it became available on the facilities market.

The provision of production technology was also altered by the activities of specialist technical service suppliers working with independent sports production companies. The Broadcasting Act of 1990 with the introduction of independent and regional production quotas had already boosted free market provision. As independent sports production companies generally lacked the capital to own expensive production equipment, so they entered commercial relationships with specialist outside broadcast facility firms and post-production houses.

For video editing, it wasn't traditional broadcasters that were on the frontline when it came to providing state-of-the-art equipment; it was often commercial post-production houses. The role of post-production houses and other technical service providers is often overlooked. Independent sports production companies now had more choice and access to the latest technology without incurring prohibitive capital costs. This market paved the way for some important innovations as digital technology was rolled out.

3.3   Digital production technology arrives

The mid-1990s was a critical period as digital production was introduced to television sport, changing work practices and output in several significant ways.

Although live broadcasts were growing in prominence, videotape remained the hub of television sports productions. But the capability of videotape was changing. From 1994 Digital Betacam enabled the entire acquisition-to-edit path to be converted to digital. In addition to higher quality and more robust video and audio signals, more creative options in editing became possible. On a practical level, cloning could be achieved without significant loss of quality and, in edit suites, source tapes could be 'pre-read' meaning a second play in machine was not needed, saving time and money.

However, the two most significant introductions were non-linear editing systems and tapeless digital media technologies. These technologies combined to (a) provide a dramatic change in sports production workflows, particularly large-scale productions, (b) revolutionise the volume and scope of sports content, including (c) the speed at which content could be produced.

In terms of non-linear editing systems, AVID became the preferred tool. Essentially AVID is a hard disk (computer) system with software that mimicked the flexibility of 16mm film editing. Content is played in from tape, or ingested. The AVID makes a virtual copy; this copy can be broken down into shorter sequences, labelled and allocated to bins from where it can be retrieved. Once in AVID content could be edited and re-edited as required. This is a non-linear and non-destructive process, so sequences can be dropped into the timeline with the remaining material pushed down the timeline (in effect extended to accommodate the new sequence) and is very different to linear videotape editing with its fixed timeline. As AVID marketing put it, producers could now 'change your mind without losing your mind'. This claim was severely tested in early AVIDs as one producer recalls:

It [AVID] was horrible. Not because it was a bad thing but because of the bugs. It was hard to do anything. It would always freeze up. (Senior sports producer, independent sport production, 2012)

New iterations of AVID offered more processing power (they got quicker) and storage for more media (they became more useful). As AVID was widely adopted a demand grew for a central storage facility, or central server, that could provide regular back up as well as shared access for multiple AVID users. The AVID Unity was that device and could serve up to 20 clients, this made it an appealing tool for host broadcast operations where multiple rights-holding broadcasters wanted to access all material as quickly as possible. This system provided a very significant breakthrough in production methods, with coverage of the World Rally Championship provided by Chrysalis Sport one of the earliest examples of AVID Unity deployment. There are three notable breakthroughs: 1) the ability to use non-linear editing to construct entire programmes, 2) *simultaneous* access to the original content for 3) *numerous* users. This meant no more copying of videotapes in real time, just plug-in with AVID, access the server and edit. Multiple output versions could now be generated from the *same original source content* as different productions worked in parallel. The increase in volume, scope and speed this provided wasn't just substantial, it was a genuine game changer.

Turning to tapeless digital media technologies, EVS is the key development. The power of EVS rests in its capacity to ingest live input from multiple sources (cameras) and to replay, and/or clip together sequences virtually *instantaneously*, without any interruptions to workflow – no action need ever be missed. Experienced directors confirm that EVS operators became essential members of the outside broadcast team. A highly respected international live sports producer describes the advent of EVS and servers:

> The tape-based environment was gone and an eight channel EVS, whilst taking up the same space as four videotape machines, was much, much more capable. If you wanted to, you could start a replay of a cricket ball being bowled *before* the delivery was actually finished... it was simply revolutionary. (International sports television director, 2012)

Another veteran live sport producer sees the development of replays in digital production as creating a major talking point among viewers:

> EVS allows you to isolate nearly every camera and to choose from around 20 different replay angles. So, when you want to review, say, a penalty incident, you have seven or eight angles ready to look at immediately. The way replays have changed is one of the single biggest step changes in sports coverage. (Live sports director, 2013)

The EVS was extremely fast and delivered multiple replays. Soon EVS servers could be linked, this meant that very large amounts of media could be moved rapidly before being played out from another EVS. Speaking in 2012 an experienced live sports director sums up the consequences: 'with digital, the scale of outside broadcast ambitions really began to increase'.

Post-2000, EVS provided media management systems using EVS Logging and IP Director software that could link a central server with a permanent archive system. Content could be pushed between locations but was still available for instant broadcast. The implications for sports production methods were enormous as, unlike transmission, sports production now had a *fully integrated digital workflow with common standards* that everyone could work with.

EVS has also had an impact on incoming feeds of live sports. An example is Sky Sports coverage of NFL, this feed has US pattern commercial breaks with internal US programme promotions and numerous sponsored segments. Sky Sports routes the incoming feed through EVS where it is delayed for up to three minutes allowing Sky Sports producers to manoeuvre their way in and out of unwanted material via their own studio presentation. The result is a presentation minus the distractions that still feels as if it is live. Typically, athletics and golf productions use EVS to 'stack' action and play back as required to tell the story of the event.

Although new digital recording formats were introduced for cameras and a range of specialist computer graphic paintboxes also developed, the introduction of AVID, central servers and EVS was by far the most significant development as new workflows offered a combination of speed, volume and scope that was radically different to the limitations of the analogue methods they replaced.

Digital broadcasting takes over

In the UK the launch of Sky Digital in 1998 was significant. Digital broadcast signals are more robust than analogue, plus improved compression methods meant that the scarcity issue with analogue frequencies was no longer relevant. With continual improvements in compression not only were there more channels but these channels could also be cheaper to operate.

A further development was high definition (HD). HD is not clearly defined; it is simply a higher definition than standard definition. According to an experienced senior Sky Sports director speaking in 2012, HD was the 'logical expression in the up-scaling in capability that digital allowed'. The director continues to explain:

> The switchover to HD was taken very seriously by Sky Sports. For example, a four-day cricket match at the Oval was used as a test bed for the entire production team, including the signal pathway from the Oval, via BT Tower and back to Sky Sports (but was not sent to air). (Sky Sports director, 2012)

Whilst the production team wondered whether they could track a fast-moving cricket ball with HD cameras, or how a presenter's make up might look under increased scrutiny, the director confirmed:

> The picture side worked out smoothly, it was in EVS/VT and sound where they had to work hardest. Sky Sports also introduced 5.1 Dolby at the same time and this had different delays compared to two-track stereo so, altogether, this was a big step up. In EVS/VT, the biggest

headache was how to incorporate an SD picture [4x3] in the HD output [16x9]. (Sky Sports director, 2012)

Since 2004–05 the adoption of digital technology has revolutionised sports production workflows; it has enabled an exponential increase in the *volume* of sport produced, it allows a wider *scope* of sports content to be made and production is *accelerated*.

3.4 Contemporary digital production technology and workflows

Digital technology facilitated a dramatic increase in sports production output – it was the extension of ways the *same original content* could be *simultaneously* re-packaged in *alternative formats* by *different users* that was pivotal in meeting the rising demand for sports content. In addition to the technological dimension, a political economy approach requires an interest in who does what and why. To help answer these questions, and to gauge the full scale of this remarkable transformation, previous analogue workflows can be compared with a contemporary case study.

Football on the frontline

In 1992 the BBC's *Match of The Day* format provided a sample workflow (see section 3.2). By the 2013–14 season a battle for the UK's live football viewers was being fought between challenger, BT Sport, and market leader BSkyB. But, away from the headlines, there is another Premier League football provider. Without attracting much media attention the Premier League operates its own production service, Premier League Productions.

Why does the Premier League offer this service? Whilst domestic rights for 2013–16 are valued at around £3 billion the international rights worth a further £2 billion (Harris, 2012), so this is an increasingly important market. Seeking to collect this revenue the Premier League controls its intellectual property according to a senior executive in charge of output speaking in 2013, 'via a guaranteed standardised and high quality output aimed at a global rather than a local (UK) audience'. The provision of this service is now discussed.

Premier League Productions (PLP)

Set up in 2004, Premier League Productions (PLP) is funded by the Premier League and operated by IMG Sports Media. PLP offers content production, distribution and archive management for the Premier

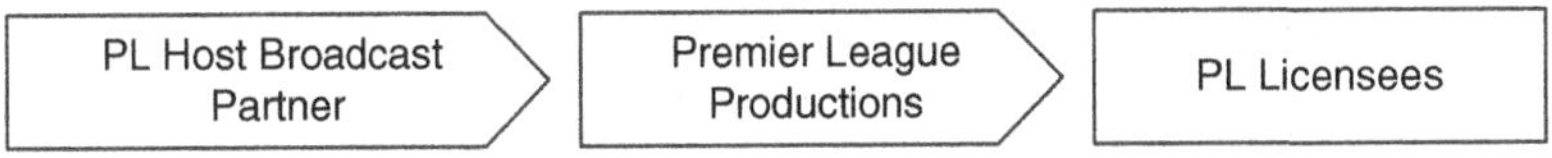

| PL Host Broadcast Partner | Premier League Productions | PL Licensees |

Figure 3.2 Host to Licensee pathway

League. According to IMG's managing director, Graham Fry, the company started working for the Premier League in 1998, 'to start with we [IMG] covered non-live matches on three cameras; three years later on just four cameras', (Gibson, 2015c).

At the start of the 2013–14 season, Premier League Productions delivered content to Premier League Licensees in 212 different territories. Using digital technologies and integrated production workflows this is a modern football content factory; the scale is unmatched by any other sports league.

What does PLP do?

Primarily, PLP takes the original match coverage provided by the Premier League's host broadcast partners, Sky Sports and BT Sport, and, with some modifications, re-broadcasts all 10 matchday fixtures across a weekend making these available to the Premier League's international Licensees.

On behalf of licensees, PLP also provides small local enhancements to this coverage, including in-vision customisation from Premier League venues. Specially enhanced feeds and multiple-match packages are also offered.

PLP produces a very high volume of content in a variety of live and pre-recorded formats, from news to classic matches. Together, the live matches, special feeds and formatted programming comprise a core production offer. According to the executive producer of PLP, Nick Moody:

> We produce a half-time and full time world feed programme. There are a number of additional properties we've added over the years: a superfeed, a multi-angle replay service, a clips channel, dedicated wide angle, a tactical feed, dedicated interview lines, all these additional things we've added as the broadcasters make more demand on us. We started with one magazine show, we now do seven a week. On average, that's 5,000 hours of content we distribute a week. (Moody, cited in Gibbons, 2015c)

Whilst there is a significant amount of duplication within the 5,000 hours this remains a bewildering array of specialist feeds. According to Fry, 'the game had completely changed' by 2007 when the value of overseas rights to the Premier League reached an estimated

£208 million a year, a significant increase from £8 million in 1992. Responding to the market, since 2010 PLP has also offered a full content service (in other words, a standalone fully scheduled channel that runs 24 hours a day seven days a week for 42 weeks each year). Via a dedicated digital department PLP also provides short-form material for www.premierleague.com.

As the domestic broadcasting rights to live Premier League football in the UK are held by Sky Sports and BT Sport, PLP's presentation of 380 games a season is exclusively focussed on the Premier League's overseas partners. If you see a Premier League match outside the UK then you will be watching PLP output.

Digital technology applied

This section explains (a) the technology used in a contemporary digital production environment and (b) how this technology has been configured to enable a remarkable increase in the volume and scope of output including the speed with which this output can be produced. This example also underlines Mosco's claim about how commodification and different outputs '...intensify the commodification process by linking increasingly specific kinds of programming to increasingly well-defined audiences' (Mosco, 1996:152).

The technology is EVS and AVID. EVS is at the hub of contemporary sport production operations, managing media at outside broadcasts and studio base. The combination of EVS technologies and software systems – including IP Logger and IP Director software – is the foundation for content logging (descriptions of content and other relevant metadata), clipping together content (a faster option than AVID editing) and the storage and movement of large amounts of media instantaneously between galleries, edit suites and MCR (MCR is the technical control area where all routing is managed).

AVID non-linear edit suites are the factory floor; the edit rooms where content is assembled before output. AVID edit bays are linked together via nearside archive systems where shared media can be accessed quickly and by multiple producers. Far side storage is a longer-term archiving solution where content is held offline and is, therefore, not available for immediate use. Typically EVS, AVID Unity and/or Viz Ardome (a media management system) are used. The key points are: 1) these systems feature a high degree of connectivity which allows large amounts of media to be moved around rapidly, 2) multiple producers can work on the same source material simultaneously, therefore 3) the volume and scope of output is dramatically increased as is 4) the speed of production. This is a quantum leap from earlier linear tape-based analogue systems. An example of how content flows from the initial match to international licensees follows.

Premier League, from stadium to international licensee

Host Broadcast Partners. The Premier League's host broadcast partners are Sky Sports and BT Sport. They are responsible for covering 154 matches a season (2013–16) for UK broadcast, with all 380 matches covered for international output. An illustrative camera plan for match coverage in the 2013–14 is set out in figure 3.3, camera positioning is subject to case-by-case restrictions imposed by individual stadia. The onward production pathway from the match, via PLP, to the licensee is illustrated in figure 3.4.

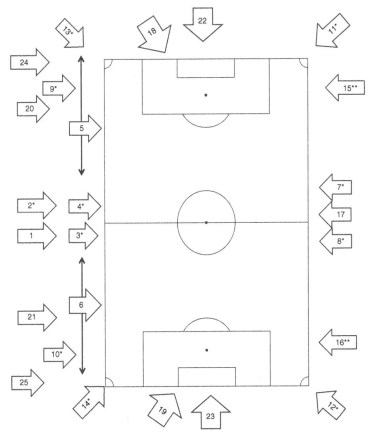

Figure 3.3 Typical HBP PL Camera Plan
20:1 lenses except, * = 86:1 (cams 9–14 with Superslo) and ** = 100:1 with Ultra Motion.

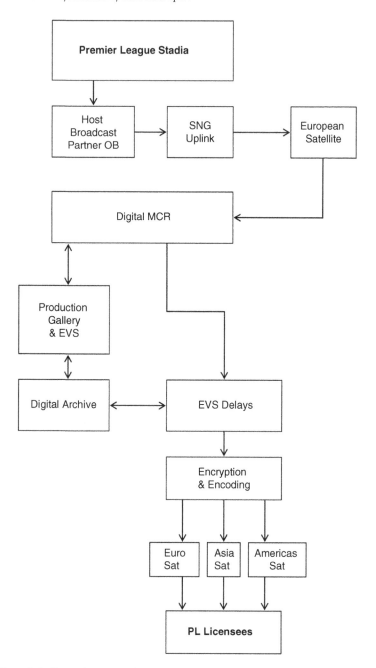

Figure 3.4   Typical PLP signal path, from PL Stadia to Licensee

Compared to the six-camera plan from 1992, often between 22–30 cameras are deployed. Six cameras provide Super Slow Motion. Two Ultra Motion cameras provide additional high levels of detail. All camera output is strictly assigned to EVS; this is done to ensure superfast replay reactions whenever called for by the director.

In a typical analogue outside broadcast truck the vision mixer console was limited to a maximum of 48 inputs, an international sports director explains the differences:

> Digital switchers [vision mixer desks] now have up to 168 inputs, eight channels of EVS is pretty standard, plus three different graphics sources are a fairly normal specification. The technological changes within a fully digital operation mean that, in the same space as older outside broadcasts, there is just so much more capability. (International sports director, 2012)

Being able to generate many more replays via EVS also means more production and/or EVS operators are required to select and manage this media. Similarly, the increased demand for statistics and graphics means either one or two assistant producers are assigned to this task. Whilst the host broadcast partner match coverage is for local UK viewers, Premier League Productions re-orients all match presentation towards a global audience. How this is done is now reviewed.

The digital production environment

Premier League Productions receives a clean feed (match coverage minus Sky Sports and BT Sport commentators, graphics and other embellishments such as station identification) from all Premier League matches covered by the host broadcast partners.

To provide a standardised high quality output of all matches, the PLP production team consists of about eight people – a director/vision mixer, two producers, two assistant producers, two EVS operators and a graphics operator. Standardised high quality output is a crucial idea that recurs in the context of UEFA, FIFA and Olympic host broadcast operations. As the match is fed into the production gallery, an assistant producer uses IP Logger software to produce a detailed description for editorial and archive use. This metadata remains attached to the media as it moves from EVS nearside storage, to the AVID, back to EVS or Ardome and then to archive. Compared to the hand-written notes made in the early 1990s (which could be of variable quality and were prone to being misplaced) IP Logger provides comprehensive data for multiple users.

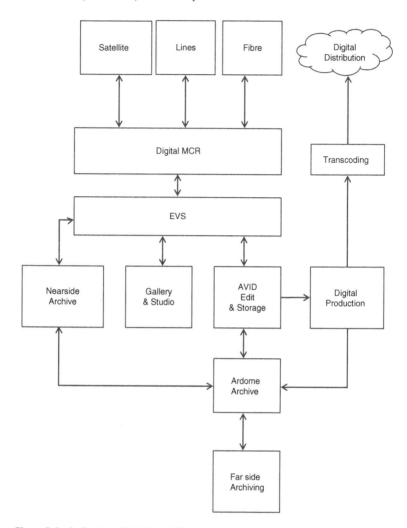

Figure 3.5   Indicative digital workflow

The 'new' output from the gallery is returned to MCR before onward routing to European, Asian and American satellite distribution and then to its final destination, with each of the 212 Premier League Licensees (figures 3.4 and 3.5).

IMG managing Director, Graham Fry, confirms the objective, 'every game looks identical. It doesn't matter whether it's QPR against Leicester or Manchester United against Liverpool, it will be treated the same and look the same' (Gibson, 2015c). The goal is consistent branding, from adding new commentaries, providing bespoke graphics for each individual element of coverage and presentation, including studios, through to generic PL logos and even the music used every new element is designed to signal 'Premier League'.

Digital production workflows

The power of digital workflows, as expressed by Doyle (2002:30), is the ability 'to reduce all sorts of images, sounds and text to a common format and to transport these via a common distribution infrastructure'. What should be added to this understanding is the ability of numerous outputs to be created *simultaneously*, hence output is *accelerated* and volume *increased*. This is the fulcrum around which sports production processes now revolve – in a sense it is a powerful digital hub that allows content to be ingested, produced, modified and re-packaged, broadcast and then archived. Looking at the Premier League, the objective is to take all matches produced locally in the UK and reversion output as an international standardised high quality presentation for use by up to 212 global licensees. In doing so, Premier League Productions delivers the Premier League brand to the world.

Turning now to the full service content service, this is simply a more structured format for content delivery, one that allows licensees to lift out and broadcast individual programmes or, if preferred, to use the schedule as a standalone channel. This option is appealing for telecommunications companies that do not have the same infrastructure as broadcasters, including production staff. The full content service includes material from the core service, but adds a range of live and pre-recorded studio programmes, plus more match re-runs and archive-based content. The full service content is a live stream; this feed is routed to a series of regional satellites, where it is available for Premier League Licensees to access. The step up to providing a full channel schedule requires a much larger volume of content (a continuous feed of 168 hours per week) plus a wider scope of programme formats.

Analysis and additional studio-based production

To provide sufficient content to fill a continuous channel PLP provides: (1) sophisticated analysis tools used as a focus for further discussion with (2) studio-based programmes providing the primary format for this expansion.

In contrast to EVS, AVID and Ardome analysis devices do not share a single operating system, meaning their incorporation is technically more challenging. However, they are important tools when adding scope to output. Of these the most notable are tOG-SPORTS Pro, the Viz-RT Touchscreen, Venatrack Real View and Red Bee Piero, licensed by the BBC.

For the 2013–14 season the Premier League introduced *Goal Decision System* from Hawkeye. Used during the match the referee is informed (via a receiver worn on the wrist) if a goal has been scored, subsequent animations can be shown on the venue screens and used in match coverage. NFL coverage has benefitted from the 1st and 10 graphics system developed by ESPN in 1998, this, and other versions, create a virtual 10 yard line illustrating how far the offense team needs to progress from the line of scrimmage to secure a first down. This enhancement has been so successful it is hard to imagine NFL coverage without it. Returning to football, there is no indication that the appetite for performance-related information is diminishing with more and more data being made available for dissection.

What is crucial here is not the technological embellishment *per se*, but the ability to recycle original media in an increasingly wide range of new programme formats. With more and more versions being generated from a limited quantity of original material the commodification process, as described by Mosco (1996) and Schimmel (2005), enters an unprecedented new level of activity. Whilst Sky Sports was the first media provider to provide significantly extended scope, this is an important development that is now being driven by the leagues and federations as they seek more control of their own output and additional revenues, particularly in international media markets. The output provided by Premier League productions provides a useful example.

3.5   Output: significantly increased volume and scope

Comparing the BBC's *Match of The Day* output from 1992 with Premier League Productions output in 2014 illustrates the remarkable increase in volume and scope that is possible using digital technology and workflows. In 1992 the weekly MoTD presentation was limited to 90 minutes. By contrast, Premier League Productions' full content service runs 24 hours a day, seven days a week devouring 168 hours of content per week, around 65 hours of which is newly produced material.

Premier League Production's output is split into 4 categories for distribution to Licensees, including:

- Core Production – a range of live and recorded programmes, plus an additional five packages featuring enhanced feeds.

- Full Content Service – a fully scheduled channel (launched in August 2010) that delivers Premier League content 24 hours a day, seven days per week, across 42 weeks per year in high definition.
- Archive-based Content – a selection of classic matches, greatest goals and golden moments from the Premier League.
- Digital Production – news feeds, press conference coverage, club guides and short features re-versioned from the core production.
- Distribution – from acquisition to multipoint distribution. Premier League Productions offer three packages with differing scales of cost and signal quality/reliability.

A brief review of each of the output categories and distribution follows.

3.5.1 Core production

Live

Beyond providing a guaranteed or uniform standard of live match production, output is extended up to 40 times per year with a super feed. This is an enhanced live offer where licensees have the option for 5–10 minutes access to their own unilateral feed (for example, to have their reporter appear in vision inside the ground before the match). Additional replays of key match incidents, as well as isolated camera angles tracking individual players are provided. The *Football Feast* feed is an extended presentation that includes up to three consecutive matches, plus a compilation of all the goals scored on a Saturday. Approximately 30 *Football Feasts* are offered per season.

Pre-recorded and magazine content

In addition to live coverage, weekly preview and review shows are offered, plus season preview and review programmes and a goals of the season compilation. There is a weekly magazine programme that focuses on lifestyle stories featuring Premier League players in the UK and from around the world, *Premier League World* offers high levels of production value and, reminiscent of the NBA's *Inside Stuff* magazine, it acts as a useful promotional tool for the Premier League.

3.5.2 Full content service

According to a senior PLP executive producer, from around 2007 there was a significant shift in the ownership of broadcasting rights:

Telecommunications corporations (Telcos) started to acquire broadcasting rights in direct competition with more conventional broadcasters. Whilst Telcos often have multiple digital broadcast platforms at their disposal, they seldom carry the support infrastructure associated with conventional broadcasters, including the technical facilities and experienced production staff to receive, make, schedule and deliver their programmes.

Although Telcos were hungry for attractive new content, many of these firms remained reluctant to undertake the financial commitment to produce their own programming to accompany their content acquisitions. (PLP executive producer, 2013)

In response to changing demand, the Premier League and PLP devised a full content service model – this is a fully structured service that runs 24 hours a day, seven days a week for 42 weeks a year. The high definition service provides licensees with content that can be aired as a standalone channel. In the 2013–14 season the channel is broadcast in South Africa and the Middle East, but in Singapore and on Sport 24 local programming is added at peak times in the schedule.

For the 2013–14 season, a typical week (168 hours) of full content Premier League service included:

- 42.5 hours of exclusive live content
- 52 hours of full match re-runs
- 22.5 hours of magazine content
- 25.5 of Premier League Archive material
- 25.5 hours of studio-based content repeats

The Premier League full content service includes core live production and archive-based content and is bolstered further by live and pre-recorded studio programmes and magazine shows. The service turns to a range of studio-based formats to fill out the schedule. The studio formats include an exclusive Premier League news service; the Premier League is the only football league that provides a 30-minute news programme, three days a week. Further studio-based formats include a matchday goals round-up service, a daily highlights/review/discussion format, including detailed analysis. There is a heavy reliance on player performance statistics and subjective player ratings.

A fanzone format includes fan access with contributors via Skype, in addition to the usual methods, such as SMS text, email, and Twitter. Fans provide a studio audience for a quiz format featuring representatives of all 20 Premier League clubs. To populate the various studio formats a substantial cast of presenters, pundits and named guests is required. The on-screen team stretches to around 30 people, including: 10 established presenters, approximately 12 football pundits and another dozen or so regular guests.

The full content service does not distribute commercial content, but commercial time (to sell advertising space) is offered to the licensees across the schedule. If licensees choose not to sell this time they can broadcast a range of interstitials, short promotions, archive clips, clips from magazine shows, picks of the week and top five/top ten lists that are provided by PLP to fill the four minute breaks.

3.5.3 Archive-based content

Since the early 1990s leagues and federations came to realise the financial value of sports media archives. In 2013–14 the Premier League Archive was managed by IMG Sports Media via a separate contract: IMG seeks to exploit potential synergies between the Premier League Archive and Premier League Productions. The PL Archive team was responsible for advising on rights values and for additional one-off sales of Premier League content in the market. However, the contract with Premier League Productions also provided access to a range of archive-based content in various formats, including classic matches.

For the core production offer, archive content includes 75 classic matches, 40 golden moments, greatest goals programmes and a format called *a whole new ball game*. Unsurprisingly, archive use is extended further for the full content service offer, where 104 classic matches are presented. *Best Classics* is another archive-based strand; these matches, sometimes featuring teams not currently in the Premier League, are broadcast over the dark weeks when there is a break in Premier League matches to accommodate international football fixtures and during the summer recess. Archive-based content accounts for just over 15% (25.5 hours) of the full service content provision.

3.5.4 Digital production

Content produced by Premier League Productions has been re-versioned for use on www.premierleague.com since 2007. The bulk of digital production is made up of: one minute news bulletins, club guides, press conference presentations and short form features. There is also an audio podcast. Speaking to executives involved, digital production is often treated like a miniaturised content operation, but with the final delivery taking different forms (e.g. encoding for use on multiple devices including Apple iOS and Android). Premier League Productions also produces Premier League content for Yahoo UK, insofar as Yahoo's Internet rights in the UK allow. This includes highlights of 380 matches, 35 matchday previews, news segments and up to six specially produced features. The preference is for short form content packaged together under a clear theme.

3.5.5 Distribution

Delivering high volumes of content to multiple points is a key element of the service. Satellite delivery is the basis of Premier League Productions' distribution operation; the large number of licensees and their global locations, taken in conjunction with the three-year cycle of broadcasting rights, underpins the practicality of delivery by satellite. Whilst some licensees may prefer file-based delivery, satellite systems remain the dominant method. As redundancy is a very costly insurance policy (redundancy is the back-up route used to ensure delivery of content, particularly for live feeds for which expensive advertising may have been sold by the licensees), so PLP uses satellite distribution to offer three levels of service based on price, quality and technology. The tiers are distinguished by preference, from extra cautious triple redundancy through to no redundancy at all. The editorial content provided remains the same for all three packages.

Premier League Productions, a new level of commodification

Measured against the BBC's 1992 edition of *Match of The Day*, the volume and scope of output now generated by Premier League Productions (PLP) from a single Premier League matchday (10 matches across a weekend) during the 2013–14 season is worth considering.

PLP's core production offer includes eight different editorial strands, from live match coverage through to studio-based programmes organised around analysis, discussion, previews and reviews. The offer also provides a further five special feed packages, with additional matches and enhancement options. On behalf of PLP, IMG has claimed it distributes an average of 5,000 hours each week of the season, (Gibson, 2015c)

The continuous feed full content service delivers a further 11 variations on output available on a channel that runs 24 hours a day, seven days of the week for 42 weeks of the year. On top of this, archive-based content and digital production deliver another four strands of programming each.

This remarkable volume – a minimum of *32 different formats* scheduled across 168 hours of broadcasting – is derived from the coverage of 10 Premier League matches across a weekend, this is a little over 900 minutes of football action (even allowing for an average of four minutes added time per game this is only 940 minutes). For every single minute of on-the-field Premier League action, Premier League Productions generates over *11 minutes of on-screen content* – a multiplication factor of 11x1. This increased output is made possible by digital technology and fully integrated production workflows.

When researchers describe a continuous expansion in the way in which (a) television can be distributed (Doyle, 2002), (b) look at how the commodification process has intensified with (c) ever more specific programmes for increasingly well-defined audiences (Mosco, 1996), or (d) how commodification is bound up in the processes of economic production and distribution (Mason, 1999) then the example of how technology has transformed the production (supply) of Premier League content is particularly revealing.

Conclusion

This chapter considered the different ways that technology has radically transformed transmission and sports television production methods.

In transmission, and against a background of changing expectations, manual videotape-based methods were replaced by automated systems utilising powerful media servers and software that was capable of scheduling and transmitting multiple channels to numerous territories and time zones at the same time. However, the transition to a fully digital and tape-free workflow in transmission was not straightforward. It was delayed due to the reliability of Digital Betacam videotape and a lack of standardised encoding standards for file-based delivery systems. This lack of standards remains problematic in transmission.

With the arrival of Sky Sports *live* coverage rapidly became the predominant style of sports broadcasting, rising to similar levels of importance found in the US. Aggressive channel marketing was also introduced. Working within the existing analogue paradigm Sky Sports escalated the amount of technology deployed for coverage. Adopting several overtly US methods Sky Sports extended Roone Arledge's philosophy of close up and personal coverage.

The arrival of digital production technology, with new workflows and faster ways of working, dovetailed perfectly into the sports television environment. It totally transformed potential output. Large volumes of media could be quickly transferred between locations but what was most revolutionary was the capacity to allow simultaneous access by numerous clients to the same original material.

Since 1992 there have been two important phases for sport production: 1) between 1994 and 2004 key non-linear editing and tapeless media technology was rolled out; introduced to production workflows this enabled a much greater volume and scope of sports content to be produced than ever before, and; 2) from 2004 onwards sports federations, including the Premier League, were able to harness the potential of new technology and workflows to produce, under their own control, a guaranteed standard or global output that closely aligned with their own brand values.

The Premier League's production arm, Premier League Productions, was unpacked and contemporary workflows and output examined, including the ways that *a single minute* of live football action is transformed into *11 minutes* of general programming for worldwide consumption via a dedicated Premier League channel. Representing a new level of intensity in the commodification process, PLP output has come a very long way from the BBC's 1992 *Match of The Day* operation.

This chapter offered a supply side explanation of television sport, including how vastly increased demand for sports content has been met. The chapter is designed to complement the demand side explanation often favoured in political economy interpretations.

In many instances developments in technology, including new distribution platforms and means of producing content, are fully expressed when new broadcasting rights are issued. As many important broadcasting rights are issued every three years then the technological paradigm is, in a sense, only updated a full three-year cycle of rights behind technological developments. The role of broadcasting rights, as the second of three influential pre-production factors, is discussed in Chapter 4.

4
Sports broadcasting rights

If Chapter 3 was concerned with fast-moving developments in technology including accelerated means of producing ever more content, then turning to a discussion of broadcasting rights means, more or less, hitting the brakes; rights are very often about what you *cannot* do as a broadcaster or producer.

Competition between broadcasters to acquire the most appealing sports broadcasting rights is extremely intense. Political economists argue that understanding why live sports coverage is so important to contemporary global media requires knowledge of how the power relations between sports authorities and broadcasters have changed over time. A strong expression of how the balance of power has shifted is seen in the process of issuing broadcasting rights. As Haynes (2005) points out:

> What is at stake is the ability of specific sports to drive uptake of new media technologies and pay-TV services. Sport, more than any other form of media content, has been used as a weapon to break into new markets, undermine competitors and ultimately dominate certain sectors of the media industry. (Haynes, 2005:6)

Evens, Iosifidis and Smith (2013:10) add: '... the marketisation of the television industry had fundamental implications for the selling and exploitation of sports broadcasting rights'. However, the story of rights is incomplete as it tends to be told with most emphasis on the demand side. Contracts for sports broadcasting rights have another, less understood dimension: the addition of increasingly detailed prescriptions from federations including UEFA, FIFA and the IOC about how sports content should be shown on screen. This trend merits examination.

As Drahos and Braithwaite (2002:4) note, such activity represents a 'quiet accretion of restrictions...' and is often hidden from the public gaze. Discussion of how increasingly prescriptive controls are added to broadcasting rights is very scarce, so the chapter is aimed at this gap.

Without advocating technological determinism, this book argues that broadcasting rights often reflect important aspects of technological change. The ways new technology and workflows combined to reshape the content supply side and meet escalating demand for sports content were examined in Chapter 3. Whilst reflecting economic and business imperatives, broadcasting rights are frequently linked to technology via new distribution platforms and means of producing content. Following intervention by competition authorities in the UK and Europe, broadcasting rights to the most popular sports events are typically tendered every three years; the majority of expert contributors interviewed thought broadcasting rights operated one cycle [of rights issued] behind technology. The pattern that emerges is of ever more specific rights being issued. This involves the unbundling of what were once more generic broadcasting rights, to be replaced with discrete categories identifying more rights, platforms, markets and territories that command further fees, for example, the introduction of overseas, Internet and mobile rights. This chapter focuses on sports broadcasting rights.

There are two dimensions to consider, (a) the ways sports broadcasting rights impact on broadcasters, and (b) how the subsequent rights contracts can go a long way to determining production output – in other words, how such contracts increasingly tell producers what to do. Again, political economy discussion has had a lot to say about the wider impact on broadcasters and the ownership of rights but has had a lot less to say about the supply side, about how broadcasting rights influence the final output that we see on television. Speaking in 2013, a widely respected sports television executive summarises:

> In terms of limiting creativity, *prescriptive* is the right word for these contracts... Is there more and more prescription in terms of what you are allowed to do and less and less input from producers? Yes. That's the case. (Executive producer, independent sport production, 2013)

For Haynes (2005) this is a story of 'the increasing use of intellectual property rights in the everyday activities of media organisations and how that has become the most important assets in media markets' (Haynes, 2005:12).

Since the mid-1990s a large part of my work as an executive producer has been responding to Requests for Production (RFP) or Invitations to Tender (ITT), processes that follow successful rights acquisitions; I have made use of this experience where non-disclosure agreements allow. In terms of contributions, it is noted that some contributors were much more reluctant to comment when the influence of leagues and federations was scrutinised, even though the contributions were anonymous. For other contributors, short form interviews that dealt with specific topics, many of which arose off the back of work situations, were used, including interrogation around the content and use of production manuals.

4.1 What is intellectual property and what is it for?

Gratton and Solberg (2007:146) argue that sports broadcasting rights serve the same purpose as copyrights do for books, films and music. However, historically there has not been any clear understanding of copyrights of sporting events. Evens, Iosifidis and Smith (2013:88), following Szymanski (2009), provide a useful summary of claims to rights ownership. As sports broadcasting rights are a form of intellectual property, the view expressed here is that ownership resides with the leagues and federations that provide the competitive context.

The ultimate structure of intellectual property regulations, such as copyright, has its roots in political philosophy; John Locke created a political philosophy of property in the seventeenth century. All patents, trademarks, design rights and rights in databases are based on intangible property rights; an example of something tangible might include a plot of land. Consequently, intellectual property rights are based on an abstract object. The World Trade Organisation suggests that intellectual property rights are given to people over the creation of the mind. However, rights are only extended to fixed, original and creative *expressions*, in other words any ideas need to be written down, as the ideas themselves are not protected. The initial idea to form a breakaway league of football clubs in England would not be protected, but the proposed new league's title (The Premier League), its constitution, playing structure, schedule of matches and other operating parameters, could be identified, set down and, at that point, would be protected. In copyright law this is known as the idea/expression dichotomy and is a source of confusion. Haynes (2005) also notes:

> Unlike tangible property, which may have clear lines of demarcation, intellectual property knows no bounds... Policing and protection of

the copying, use and exploitation of IP rights is therefore a key mechanism for society – largely led by business interests – to demarcate who owns what. (Haynes, 2005:14)

Once you own an intellectual property, the next step is to attach a value. The original owner holds various rights to copy until they are assigned to someone else, either by being sold or licensed. The bundle of rights that can, according to Haynes (2005:17), be assigned includes reproduction, derivative works adaptation or translation, broadcast, and public performance. These are the *primary* rights. *Secondary* rights protect against secondary infringement of copyright and include unauthorised distribution and exploitation of copied, importation, rent for hire, exhibiting for public trade, and selling. For example, a UK broadcaster may have the right to show Premier League football, but these primary rights would not allow the broadcaster to sell their coverage on to a third party, a foreign broadcaster, as this would require a secondary rights deal. In the initial (1992) Premier League broadcasting rights deal BSkyB added £30 million for the overseas rights (Horsman, 1997). For the period 2013–16 broadcasting rights for Premier League overseas sales were worth close to £2 billion (Harris, 2012), unsurprisingly the Premier League actively protects its intellectual property rights. Utilitarian, market-driven principles of copyright (as they are interpreted by contemporary global media companies) have increasingly become the *de facto* understanding of how media rights are valued, organised and distributed. This suggests that much of copyright law is arbitrary and is designed on behalf of powerful interests.

4.2   How has copyright law developed and how it is connected to the market?

Whilst media markets have expanded globally (as has their protection under intellectual property law) there is no such thing as a homogenised international copyright and individual nation states therefore have their own histories of copyright legislation. Numerous international agreements have attempted to iron out disparities and divergences around the world. Haynes (2005:22) reviews the Berne Convention (1886), the Universal Copyright Convention (agreed under UNESCO in 1952), the foundation of the World Intellectual Property Organisation (WIPO in 1967) and Trade Related Property Rights (TRIPS agreed under GATT 1994). Where the World Intellectual Property Organisation (WIPO) acts as a secretariat for global intellectual property conventions, the World

Trade organisation (WTO) carries powerful economic remedies and sanctions over nations that fail to meet the minimum standards for Trade Related Intellectual Property Rights (TRIPS). As Herman and McChesney (1997:51) note, 'along with pharmaceuticals, media and computer software copyright are the primary topics for global intellectual property rights negotiations'.

Considering intellectual property, three factors stand out:

- Individual states sanction and regulate rules by which intellectual property rights operate; regulations vary from country to country.
- The growth in importance of intellectual property rights (including their definition and control) has been heavily influenced by the organisations that have promoted the virtues of free trade and non-interference of governments, in other words WTO, GATT and NAFTA and the EC.
- IP Rights are invariably vested in large transnational corporations whose economic power often translates into political and cultural power. Recent trends in IP rights are often concerned with what *cannot* be done and this, as Haynes (2005:10) notes, means IP rights are used to 'actually inhibit innovation and creativity'.

Haynes (2005:13) continues to argue that intellectual property rights serve the interests of transnational corporations and the global business elite. Why such intellectual property rights exist in their present form, and what they protect, reveals how their meaning and function are changing to benefit the few (owners) over the wider (public) interest (this also appears to be linked to the transformation of citizens into consumers). Sports broadcasting rights were, for Rupert Murdoch and News Corporation, a battering ram forcing entry into new markets following the deregulation (in the UK, the 1990 Broadcasting Act). The goal was to dominate global TV sport rights ownership. It has proved a successful technique in the UK with BSkyB's coverage of Premier League and in the US with Fox's presentation of the NFL.

Linked to media regulation, international treaties governed by the World Intellectual Property Organisation (WIPO) and the World Trade Organisation (WTO) have influenced developments in copyright that are contained in directives by the European Union, adopted by the UK in 2003 in what might be loosely termed as a trickle-down effect of policy from a global to a national context (see Copyright Designs and Patent Act, 1988; Copyright Related Rights Regulations, 2003). This brief discussion demonstrates that the world of intellectual property is often confusing and there is little evidence that it is getting any easier to understand. Two further factors add complication: (a) the Internet, the ease with which material can be copied and exchanged threatens the copyright control of global media providers, and; (b) the way encryption on digital delivery systems has been used to lock out users. This is known as the copyright grab whereby copy-circumvention and access-circumvention have been bundled together in digital rights management technology to limit fair use. Copyright law does not have any bearing in access provisions, so this debate will continue.

4.3   Sports broadcasting rights, changing values and definitions

As Szymanski (2006:149) points out, the television industry consists of a set of vertically related markets. 'The nature of competition at each stage of the television industry, like any other, is determined by the nature of technology.'

The first sign that the long-running arrangement between the BBC and ITV (that suppressed the value of sports broadcasting rights) was ending came in 1979 when London Weekend Television bid £5 million for exclusive rights to show league football. The press dubbed the attempted highjack of the BBC's flagship show, *Match of The Day*, as 'snatch of the day'. It was in 1988, with broadcasting deregulation on the horizon, that the cost of domestic UK broadcasting rights to football began to escalate with ITV bidding £44 million for 18 matches per season for four seasons. As Gratton and Solberg (2007:5) summarise, in 1992 BSkyB raised ITV's 1988 offer by 250% and, when the rights were renegotiated in 1997, tabled a further 337% rise in rights fees. Economically, the ownership of Premier League rights remains central to BSkyB strategy.

Valuing and Auctioning Broadcasting Rights

How do broadcasters evaluate their bids for sports broadcasting rights? Gratton and Solberg (2007) note that sports programming:

> ... almost uniquely has this ability to attract the size and characteristics of audiences most attractive to distributors, sponsors and advertisers. These audiences were also willing to pay a premium price to broadcasters to receive more of the sports content than had previously been supplied by the old free-to-air channels. (Gratton and Solberg, 2007:10)

However, Gerrard (2006:31) argues that, 'sports media and image rights are intangible assets and invariably there are severe valuation problems'. Among the drivers that shape sports broadcasting rights values are:

- The size and purchasing power of the population in the viewing market.
- The popularity of the sport among the general audience.
- The quality of the tournament, playing talent, uncertainty of outcome and contest significance.
- The type of media coverage offered.
- The level of competition on the demand side.

Haynes (2005) also reminds us that:

> Sport is ready made for television. Its use by television adds an important dimension to media rights, because how we value sport in society has a direct effect on the licensing, acquisition, distribution and ultimate consumption of sport. (Haynes, 2005:67)

A very high barrier of confidentiality, legal process and regulatory requirements surrounds the auctioning of broadcast rights by organisations such as the Premier League. Detailed information on rights, on the valuation and submission of bids and of the subsequent contracts issued are fiercely guarded.

Premier League UK broadcasting rights

Working with specialist media, business and commercial, legal and regulatory advisors leagues and federations define the broadcasting rights to their events by considering:

1) The *range* of programme packages offered, from live coverage, delayed presentation, highlights and clip rights including availability (broadcast times) for each package.
2) The *distribution* platform, including digital satellite and cable (usually pay-TV), terrestrial broadcast (free-to-air), Internet streaming and mobile. This may include further definitions such as anytime and anywhere options defined by platform.
3) The *broadcast territory*, usually defined as domestic (UK) or overseas (in the case of the Premier league this becomes 212 different territories)

4) The *period of the license*, this is now typically three years but varies, most obviously with quadrennial events including the Olympics and World Cup Finals.

Leagues, federations and their advisors consider all areas that can be exploited by the sale of their rights. Domestic rights have been the most valuable, but overseas rights have risen dramatically in recent years. Revenue from Internet and mobile rights remains modest. Live audio-visual UK broadcasting rights to the Premier League have, since 2001, been sold in three year/season licenses. The number of matches offered for live broadcast has increased from 60 (1992–97) to 154 (2013–16) and will rise again to 168 (2016–19).

The Premier League offered 154 live matches between 2013–16. Correlating several sources shows seven packages structured A to G, with each package distinguished by the time at which matches are broadcast (table 4.1). The Premier League sells the broadcasting rights of all member clubs on a collective basis. Revenue from domestic rights sales is divided on a 50:25:25 basis; 50% is shared equally between all 20 clubs: 25% is awarded on a merit basis determined by each

Table 4.1   PL Broadcasting Rights Values 2013–2016

Pack*	Purchaser	Matches	Picks**	Cost	Cost per match
A	BT	Sat 12.45	13 × 1 & 13 × 4	£534m	£6.85m
B	BSkyB	Sat 17.30 (Some matches rescheduled to Sunday 13.30)	22 × 3 & 4 × 5	£465m	£5.96m
C	BSkyB	Sun 13.30	13 × 2 & 13 × 3	£495m	£6.35m
D	BSkyB	Sun 16.00	20 × 1 & 6 × 4	£642m	£8.23m
E	BSkyB	Mon 20.00 (Some on Sun 16.00)	12 × 2 & 10 × 4 & 4 × 5	£480m	£6.65m
F	BSkyB	Sat 17.30	8 × 2 & 4 × 4	£196m	£5.5m
G	BT	2 × Sat 12.45 Plus midweek evening 17.45	5 × 1 & 5 × 2 & 2 × 5	£204m	£5.67m
				£3.018bn	

* Packs A through E offer 26 matches per pack, F and G just 12 matches per pack = 154 matches.

** There are 5 rounds of match picks; this indicates which broadcaster has the right to choose preferred matches and when. For example, for 1st round match picks BSkyB has 20 picks and BT has 18.

Sources: The Guardian, The Telegraph and Daily Mail.

club's final league position and the final 25% is distributed as a facilities fee for the matches involving any club shown live on television. For 2013–16 the championship-winning club is expected to earn close to £100 million in broadcast earnings each season, while the bottom club can expect £63 million (Ziegler, 2013). Additional revenue, the income generated from selling Premier League broadcasting rights overseas – approximately £2 billion for 2013–16 – is divided equally between the 20 premier league clubs. The average cost paid per match for domestic UK broadcasting rights has escalated from around £630,000 to £6.53 million. This represents a ten-fold increase in rights fees since 1992.

Breaking down the 2013–16 UK domestic rights:

- BSkyB purchased five packages, comprising 116 matches for a total of £2.28 billion in rights fees.
- BT Sport purchased two packages, comprising 38 matches for £738 million.

In recent years the value of overseas rights has also risen sharply. Table 4.2 shows overseas rights as an additional revenue source (except for the entry in 1992–97 which is extrapolated from the figure for overseas rights that was added to BSkyB's final offer).

Table 4.2 Rising PL Broadcasting Rights Values

Period	Duration	Domestic UK£	Purchaser	+ Overseas UK£
1992–1997	5 years	£304m	BSkyB | 60 matches	£30m
1997–2001	4 years	£743m	BSkyB | 60 matches	£98m
2001–2004	3 years	£1.2bn	BSkyB | 106 matches	£178m
2004–2007	3 years	£1.024bn	BSkyB | 138 matches	£325m
2007–2010	3 years	£1.706bn	BSkyB | 92 matches Setanta | 46 matches	£625m
2010–2013	3 years	£1.78bn	BSkyB | 115 matches ESPN | 23 matches	£1.4bn
2013–2016	3 years	£3.018bn	BSkyB | 116 matches BT Sport | 38 matches	≥£2bn
2016–2019	3 years	£5.14bn	BSkyB | 126 matches BT Sport | 42 matches	

Sources: Premier League, The Guardian, The Telegraph and Daily Mail.

In summary, from 2001–04, three packages of rights were offered and rights were issued every three years. BSkyB won the majority of matches, NTL secured pay-per-view rights and ITV won highlights rights. As NTL could not afford its offer it withdrew its bid.

For 2004–07, four packages were auctioned and BSkyB won all four. Pressure from the EU Competition Commission saw BSkyB attempt to sublicense eight games but the agreed reserve price was not met and rights reverted to BSkyB.

EU pressure paved the way for the 2007–10 license when six packages were offered, with no single bidder being able to secure all six (European Commission, 2005). This allowed Setanta to become the first broadcaster other than BSkyB to broadcast live Premier League matches. BSkyB's domination was ended by the EU Competition Commission, rather than via free market competition. In terms of further revenue for UK-based rights, the BBC paid £105m (2004–07), £172m (2007–10) and £173m (2013–16) to secure highlights rights for *Match of The Day*. From 2007, additional costs were raised for the rights to show delayed coverage – the Sky Sports match broadcast in full at 20.00 on a Saturday night, followed by 50 minute highlights of each BSkyB game at 22.15. UK Internet and mobile rights have been added recently, as an ex-Sky Sports executive speaking in 2013 confirmed, 'It was only six years ago [2007] that mobile broadcasting rights appeared for the first time'.

In February 2015 the 2016–19 UK domestic rights were awarded with the total value reaching £5.14 billion for 168 live matches, with the average value per game increasing by 70% to more £10 million. BSkyB will pay more than £11 million per game for 126 matches (£4.176 billion), whilst BT will pay £7.6 million per game for 42 matches (£738 million). BSkyB and BT will also show Friday night football for the first time (Gibson, 2015a).

Reviewing the growth of the Premier League's domestic broadcasting rights, the explosion in value of rights licensed for top-flight football in the UK is not unique. It can be argued that the increases for Premier League broadcasting rights echoed the dramatic increases in rights fees paid for NFL coverage in the US in the 1970s and 1980s. Since the 1960s it has been the NFL that has set the benchmark for broadcasting rights income. It can also be noted that the success of the Premier League, as a rival set up to challenge the incumbent Football League, was not guaranteed as, historically, in professional sports the single dominant league always prevails (Fort, 2006:150). The risk involved in the newly formed BSkyB-Premier League axis is often overlooked.

Overseas broadcasting rights

As discussed in Chapter 2, the NBA was actively engaged in building overseas rights values during the 1990s. The NBA borrowed heavily from advertising and branding cultures to create a global phenomenon around televised basketball and its leading player, Michael Jordan. Securing significant revenue from overseas rights sales was not entirely new and NBA activities were certainly well known to the Premier League. As shown in table 4.3 the revenues raised by the Premier League for its overseas distribution shows growth that roughly doubles with each period of rights:

Table 4.3 Overseas revenue for Premier League rights

1992–1997	£30 million
1997–2001	£98 million
2001–2004	£178 million
2004–2007	£325 million
2007–2010	£625 million
2010–2013	£1.2 billion
2013–2016	≥UK£2 billion

Sources: Premier League, The Guardian, The Telegraph and Daily Mail.

Recalling Fort (2006:53) and how earnings from broadcasting rights have altered the revenue side of sport forever, for 2013–16 the Premier League anticipates total rights revenues to reach £5.5 billion (Harris, 2012). With domestic rights for 2016–19 topping £5.14 billion, revenues from overseas sales are also expected to escalate. But where does the spiralling cost of sports broadcasting rights leave broadcasters?

Escalating costs

Reasons for the escalation in the value of broadcasting rights include:

- The supply of broadcasting rights to elite sports is less than the demand from broadcasters. The number of competing media providers increased substantially from 1992, whilst the number of attractive sports events has remained relatively fixed.
- Live sports programmes are *perishable goods* they cannot be stored without losing most of their value. The high degree of time sensitivity of sport represents a major difference from other entertainment products.
- Similarly, exclusivity is particularly important as rights lose value once there is no longer uncertainty over the result. However,

exclusive delayed broadcast rights and highlights rights do retain some value.

- The many ways sports coverage can be used on television, including live coverage, highlights programmes, rolling news bulletins, previews and promotions and nostalgia programmes featuring archive content, adds an important dimension to broadcasting rights. Premier League Productions, via its dedicated channel, produces 11 minutes of content for every single minute of football played on the pitch.
- The ways sports coverage can be adapted for distribution on alternative platforms, such as Internet streaming and mobile consumption is becoming more significant culturally but is not yet financially rewarding.
- In a fragmented broadcasting landscape, live coverage of major sports events continues to attract very large audiences (including audience demographics that strongly appeal to advertisers and sponsors).
- Sport is one of the few programme genres that television audiences have demonstrated they are prepared to pay to watch.
- There is a lack of viable substitutes for live sports coverage.
- However, sport does have a finite value as the crash of ITV Digital in 2002, and the failure of Premier League rights holders Setanta and the diminished profile of ESPN all demonstrate.

Broadcasting rights, the buyer's perspective

Jeanrenaud and Kesenne (2006) argue the amount broadcasters are willing to pay for premium sports rights cannot solely be explained by what they are able to earn from subscription fees, sponsorship and advertising revenues.

> By showing the most popular sports, broadcasters expect to benefit in terms of better image and identity, a stronger market position and a sustained increase in viewers. (Jeanrenaud and Kesenne, 2006:2)

The most prestigious events are the live global mega-events such as the IOC Olympics and the FIFA World Cup Finals. These marquee events provide a broadcaster with a degree of prominence that has value; in the UK, the BBC gains status as the Olympics broadcaster and, in the US, NBC's long-term association with the Olympics provides a similar benefit. But there are several issues with such rights: 1) rights to these global events can be purchased by competing sports rights agencies, for example Infront (formerly the Kirch Group), Sportfive and TEAM

Marketing before being marketed to national broadcasters territory by territory, 2) The Olympic Games and World Cup Finals are staged every four years (although, from 1992, the summer and winter Olympics were placed two years apart) and, 3) audience ratings are often determined by the performance of national athletes or, for the World Cup, the national team; when local interest is eliminated, then viewing figures tend to diminish and the value of advertising slots decrease.

As broadcasters seek to build their audiences, it is the ability of national leagues and federation-based competitions to offer popular, talent-led, high-quality sports contests, with matches played week in and week out, across a well-defined schedule that are the most highly valued and subsequently attract the highest rights fees. BSkyB has consistently used first mover strategy to secure important rights. Sky Sports MD, Barney Francis maintains: 'The Premier League has never been more popular with our customers', (www.premierleague.com, 2012). Football continues to be used to drive take up of new services, for example Sky Go, and prompted BSkyB to increase the average rights fee it paid per Premier League game from £6.5 million to more than £11 million.

In comparison to league football, the value of Formula 1 Grand Prix rights is less due to the varying start times of races; races are not held every week and frequently involve significant time shifts due to the different international time zones in a Formula 1 season. The relative uncertainty of when F1 races will be available to broadcast is slightly less appealing to audiences, advertisers and sponsors. Illustrating this point, by March 1998 the BBC had lost all its football coverage, including *Match of The Day* and was looking for another flagship sport. UEFA Champions League coverage was ruled out, as the BBC could not broadcast the embedded sponsorship. Meanwhile, at ITV, executives were keen to placate their advertisers by opting out of their contract to show Formula 1 and secure UEFA Champions League coverage. The appeal of regular mid-week prime time slots provided by elite European football outweighed the confusing schedule of F1 races. ITV was happy to openly admit this (Gibson, 2008). The BBC stepped in to secure F1 coverage. As Haynes (2005:68) argues, 'Sports rights can be, and usually are, the flagship and distinguishing factor of a television station's brand identity, and are lost at their peril'. In the case of the BBC, its inability to monetise the most expensive rights, via subscriptions, sponsorship or advertising is an economic disadvantage that is increasingly hard to overcome in a competitive market.

Moving away from elite sports, broadcasting rights for local or less popular sports can still provide value. Broadcasters can acquire advertising-funded coverage of some niche sports free of charge.

Table 4.4 provides illustrative categories set out by perceived value, by region and reach, rather than by the actual rights fees paid. Whilst it is subjective, this list demonstrates the difference between prominent sporting events that act like special offers attracting viewers to a broadcaster's schedule every four years and the regular menu of domestic leagues and federation-run competitions, with schedules that provide volume and quality across a well-defined season, that run year after year, are proven to deliver viewers and appeal to advertisers and sponsors.

In general terms, broadcasters engage with federations selling rights in the following steps:

- When a league or federation auctions its domestic broadcasting rights a confidential tender document is circulated to interested parties. (Occasionally, interested parties are invited to request a tender document alongside signature of a non-disclosure agreement to cover the tender process).
- A deadline is set for broadcasters to submit first round sealed bids for the various rights they may wish to purchase.
- Once bids are received, broadcasters may be required to make a presentation to the league or federation.
- A set of clarifications may be requested and circulated.
- In larger and more complicated tenders second round bids may be required.
- There is usually a small window for exclusive negotiation between the leagues or federations and the preferred bidder.
- The auction winners are announced 'subject to contract'.

Rights auctions are a time-consuming and increasingly expensive process for bidders; costs cannot be recovered if a bid fails. As bids require specialist commercial, financial and legal input then costs quickly mount up. In 2012, BT Sport successfully bid for two Premier League packages (38 matches). Within sports television this success is credited to the additional input of Tony Ball, a former BSkyB chief executive who worked closely with Vic Wakeling at Sky Sports. Ball was hired by BT as a non-executive director and brought first-hand experience and strategic insight to the Premier League rights bidding process. BT Vision also called on Marc Watson, its own chief executive (Sweney, 2012). Previously Watson had been a director at the sports rights consultancy firm

Table 4.4 Illustrative categories for sports rights

Global Mega Events	IOC Summer Olympic Games FIFA World Cup Finals IOC Winter Olympic Games
Global Events with secondary appeal	Various World Championships (e.g. IAAF athletics, swimming, gymnastics, rowing, sailing and so on) Rugby World Cup Finals Cricket World Cup Finals Paralympics, Summer and Winter
Regional Events with significant global appeal	The EURO Championships Copa America (South American national championships) NFL SuperBowl & AFC/NFC Conference Finals UEFA Champions League EUROPA League Formula 1 Grand Prix Moto GP (motorcycle racing) USPG and ETP men's professional Golf circuits ATP Tennis Tour 6 Nations Rugby Union
Regional Events, with less widespread appeal	World Rally Championships Federation-based football tournaments, national and club-level – e.g. Liberatores Cup Asian Games Commonwealth Games Heineken European Cup (Rugby Union) Southern hemisphere international rugby tournaments
National Leagues & competitions with significant global appeal and that provide regular season-long schedules	Premier League (UK) FA Cup (UK) La Liga (Spain) Serie a (Italy) Bundesliga (Germany) NFL (USA) NBA (USA)
National leagues & competitions with less global appeal	Horse racing – both flat and hurdles seasons League-based rugby union Super League – rugby league County cricket Major League Baseball Major League Hockey
Highlights-based content	MoTD (BBC PL football highlights magazine) BBC The Football League Show (Highlights) Recycled sports preview/review programmes (e.g. Goals on Sunday, Sky Sports)

Table 4.4   (Continued)

	Assorted magazine programmes made by both broadcasters and federations (e.g. FIFA Futbol Mundial Football, UEFA Champions League Magazine) and independent magazines, such as TransWorld Sport
Special cases	Rolling sports news (e.g. Sky Sports News)
Sponsored content	Many niche and extreme sports are funded by brands and/or sponsors and aired for free, e.g. Channel Four Freesports.
Archive-based content	Recycled nostalgia-based programmes
Sports Entertainment	Trace Sports, lifestyle-based content

Source: author's notes.

Reel Enterprises, a long-standing advisor to the Premier League in rights negotiations. Adding detailed inside knowledge of processes and politics appears to be a critical component of successful rights bids.

Production services auctions

When a broadcaster does secure broadcasting rights there may follow a further tender process, a Request for Production (RFP) or an Invitation to Tender (ITT). This is where a broadcaster, for a variety of reasons including meeting regional production quotas, may wish to place the production with an independent producer to deliver the final content. These responses can also be expensive to produce, costs are seldom recovered and I have seen cases where the tender operator seeks to retain ownership of *any* ideas submitted, even if the tender is not successful and no costs are paid. Whilst it might be argued that this is an abuse of market power I am not aware of any example where an independent production company has provided a challenge.

Rights holding federations may also wish to tender directly with an independent production company for coverage and subsequent distribution of an event. In responding to tenders I have noticed a trend for more legalistic terms to be used. As some of these events are relatively small, then production companies may take a view on whether a limited opportunity may lead to further, more lucrative work in future. As federations adopt legal frameworks the situation is reminiscent of Harvey (2005:3) and the 'significance of [extending] contractual relations in the marketplace'.

Risk, the broadcasters' dilemma

As competition has propelled the value of broadcasting rights, the risks associated with acquiring expensive rights have also increased. Since 1992 only five companies have owned live broadcasting rights for the Premier League; two of these companies have failed. When Setanta lost one of the two packages (of 23 games each) it had acquired as a result of EU intervention, the company failed to meet its commercial targets and collapsed in June 2009 (Mason and Moore, 2009). Within a few weeks ESPN acquired Setanta's rights but was unable to hold onto these rights in 2012 due to intense competition from newcomer BT Sport, since then ESPN has had a diminished profile in the UK. BT Sport began to broadcast in the 2013–14 season, so whether its acquisitions (from 2013 of two packages totalling 38 games for £738 million, and from 2016 of another two packages totalling 42 games for £960 million) is successful as more than a service designed to drive take up of its broadband services remains to be seen, leaving BSkyB as the only company with a long-term track record in monetising its ownership of domestic UK rights to live Premier League matches.

When considering sports broadcasting rights broadcasters' evaluation needs to account for the full costs incurred, from buying rights to delivering programmes to audiences. Solberg (2006:108) explains the cost structure of sports broadcasting:

- Total costs = fixed costs + variable costs
- Fixed costs = production related costs + sunk costs (usually including broadcasting rights fees and infrastructure costs)
- Variable costs = variable costs of broadcasting + variable costs of production + opportunity costs

Solberg (2006) also recognises the very different outcome from a contract that *obliges* the purchaser to broadcast a fixed number of games – the case with the Premier League – and a contract that *allows* a broadcaster to air up to (but not necessarily all of) the games offered. As BSkyB in particular has invested heavily in acquiring attractive football rights and in their broadcasting infrastructure, then there is a much higher degree of sunk costs. As Solberg (2006) continues, among other things this has allowed sellers to dictate the contract terms leaving the broadcasters to carry the entire risk in the event of negative shifts in demand – of an audience switching off. Running a commercial sports broadcasting business, even when rights fees are discounted, is extremely expensive and represents a very high barrier to entry. Whilst not referring to the acquisition of expensive sports broadcasting rights, the element of risk implied in the term *casino capitalism* (Strange, 1986) seems an appropriate description. However, the right sport can deliver large numbers of viewers to broadcasters.

With the shift in market power away from broadcasters upstream to the leagues and federations there is another, largely unseen but significant trend: the detailed prescriptions that are increasingly written in to broadcasting rights and that frequently determine key aspects of production output and that remind us, again, of 'a quiet accretion of restrictions...' (Drahos and Braithwaite, 2002:4).

4.4 Broadcasting rights and prescriptive practices, examples from Formula 1 and the UEFA Champions League

Formula 1

In 1995, ITV won the rights to broadcast live Formula 1 offering Formula 1 Management £60 million for four seasons from 1997. ITV retained the broadcasting rights until 2009. Following its acquisition, ITV tendered a Request for Production (RFP) to its own production division, ITV Sport, plus IMG and a broadcaster-independent producer partnership of Meridian, Anglia and Chrysalis Television (MACh 1). Working at Chrysalis Television, I was lead author of the successful MACh 1 response.

Formula 1 (F1) was already known for draconian arrangements at its venues, for example *any* material shot at an F1 circuit belongs to F1 – copies of all material had to be submitted on a daily basis. However, the Formula 1 contract with ITV went further in prescribing what could and could not be done at any venue. This was in 1996–97 and, whilst I had encountered copyright issues when working on behalf of Channel Four with the NFL and NBA in the US, this was the first time I had seen such extensive restrictions. Typical conditions determined:

- What material producers could record at any F1 venue.
- Whether a studio position would be allowed at any venue.
- Where any additional cameras could be placed on site, including a tight restriction on the radio (RF) frequencies used.
- When material could be recorded at the venue.
- When a rights holding broadcaster *must* use the international feed.
- Prescriptions on what could be done in and out of commercial breaks.
- How additional material, like interviews with drivers that had left the race, may be incorporated within live coverage (the international feed).

- Who producers could have access to at the venue.
- Where production (OB) vehicles could be parked.
- What levels of credentials would be authorised and who could receive them.
- What supporting F1 Archive would be available and how this could be used.
- The ownership of all material shot at the venue.
- When the final programme material can be aired, or rebroadcast on other ITV channels.

ITV was keen to make Formula 1 coverage as widely accessible as possible so the broadcaster could maximise the value of the broadcasting rights, a specific concern was to minimise the impact of commercial breaks during coverage. Additionally, producers had to balance the stipulations set out by their client, ITV with its commercial targets and audience requirements, and those set by Formula 1 – the production team was stuck in the middle between the broadcaster-client and the rights holders. A senior executive producer with many years' experience of Formula 1 coverage at different broadcasters confirmed the issues remained much the same when interviewed in 2013:

> Formula 1 limits creative control massively. Bernie Ecclestone says: this is how we cover the start of the race, half way through lap two we will do seven or eight replays of the start. This is incredibly frustrating, because halfway through lap two we haven't really resolved where this and that driver are in the race yet. But the rules that have been laid down by Formula 1 are that halfway through lap two you *must* have these replays – it is incredibly frustrating. There is now much more of a set pattern in the way that a sport is covered as a result of the requirements of rights holders. Formula 1 is a good example. (Executive producer, independent sports production, 2013)

Formula 1 was one of the first federations to actively seek a guaranteed quality of coverage across all its events; the Premier League later expressed a similar target for its own international output. A highly experienced international sport director adds his perspective on the balance between offering safety or creativity in live coverage:

> When you are directing a generic world feed to over 100 countries, it is more important to be a safe pair of hands as the premise is guaranteed uniform and stable coverage of the event. The coverage needs to be clean, so any client can jump in and out of the coverage where

they need to. You might need more creativity when you are working for a single channel – a broadcaster – because you are then responsible for how the channel looks and feels, but you don't need this creativity for an international feed. (International live sports director, 2012)

My experience of Formula 1 tallies with the accounts of several specialist F1 producers and directors interviewed. What Formula 1 had found was this: as F1 broadcasting rights were sold to more broadcasters around the world: (a) the different emphasis placed on coverage by each national Grand Prix host broadcaster was becoming increasingly incongruous as they tended to focus on local stories, teams and drivers, and (b) with increased rights sales, more broadcasters wanted to be able to drop in and out of an international feed to which they could add their own unilateral material (customising presentation for their own audiences). Either way, F1 wanted more consistent and uniform coverage from race to race and across the entire season of races – the aim was to establish a recognised F1 *brand*. This was not just editorial it was also technical due to different recording standards used around the world. However, the needs of an emerging, globalised audience had become more important than the domestic interests and idiosyncrasies of coverage from, say, the British, Italian or Brazilian Grand Prix.

To achieve greater consistency in race coverage Formula 1 provided its own host broadcast (international) feed. This feed starts five minutes prior to the start of the race lasting through to the post-race press conference. Formula 1 broadcasting rights agreements required *all* broadcasters to join this feed before the race.

Another reason for such prescriptions was to ensure that the coverage provided positive exposure for the key sponsors, whether it is those sponsoring the race, those with prominence around the circuit, or a balance of car sponsors to be shown across a full race weekend.

Between 1996 and 2002 Formula 1 went a step further and provided its own coverage from a state-of-the-art production complex at each venue. Although this coverage was innovative, it was not a commercial success. Consequently, Formula 1 entered a two year joint-venture with BSkyB gaining access to the Sky platform where it offered a digital service for £12 per race. Whilst the service added a number of engaging editorial enhancements – including a lap counter, car-tracking graphics, on-screen rev counters, G-force indicators and more team radio feeds – commercial success remained elusive. However, a positive legacy of this service is how many of these editorial enhancements were subsequently adopted in the current international feed (Milmo, 2002).

Prescriptive coverage

During interviews some producers, particularly those with more international experience, said they considered production standards around the globe had gradually improved since about 2000; in particular, standards in Asia and China showed the greatest improvement. These producers considered this was a result of exposure to prescriptive coverage required by Formula 1, FIFA and the IOC. It was argued that, in a sense, these prescriptions offered a benchmark for international standards.

During the same interviews, the most prevalent view expressed was how producers considered their own creativity had been curtailed by the same increase in prescriptive conditions. These conditions were being added much further upstream, usually at the same time as broadcasting rights were assigned. In other words, long before producers became involved. A senior executive at an independent sports production company expressed concern about the future course of this trend:

> Production creativity will be much more focussed around shoulder programming, those shows pre-kick-off and post-match, that's where producers will have input, once you go across to the stadium or race track coverage will be more prescriptive. (Senior manager, independent production, 2013)

An increase in prescriptive conditions marks a split between international *coverage*, increasingly provided by federations, and more localised *presentation* added by rights holding broadcasters. While Formula 1 was one of the earliest examples of a federation exercising control over the final production output, a landmark case illustrating how prescriptions have become formalised is found with the UEFA Champions League.

UEFA Champions League

Coverage of the UEFA Champions League (UCL) involves matches played at the same time at different locations across Europe, so similar issues of consistency of coverage and the protection of brand values arise as with Formula 1. The UCL season comprises 16 matchdays, including the final and the UEFA Super Cup. The vast majority of matches kick off at 20:45 Central European Time and are played on a Tuesday or Wednesday; the Final is on a Saturday. A head of programmes speaking in 2013 had a simple view of the issue: 'German TV would use one wipe and Austrian TV another and ITV yet another and it wouldn't look like it is all part of the Champions League family'. However, the issues in play are more complex.

Sugden and Tomlinson (1998:93–97) note UEFA worked closely with TEAM Marketing AG, a company set up in 1991 to secure 'the greatest monetary gain through marketing of television rights and sponsorship of the UEFA Champions League'. This approach reflected models created for the 1984 Los Angeles Olympics and Patrick Nally's influential *InterSoccer* template discussed in Chapter 2 (Nally, 1979).

For UEFA and TEAM Marketing the solution was to create the UEFA Champions League Production Manual. When a broadcaster acquires the rights to broadcast the UEFA Champions League it must abide by the rules set out in the Production Manual. It is telling that, when approaching the subject of federation control, many producers were reluctant to say anything critical, even when speaking with anonymity. As the focus is on prescription, the following account uses contributor interviews from practising producers and off-air analysis to interpret the UEFA Champions League Production Manual.

The UEFA Champions League Production Manual (UEFA, 2011) gets a little larger each season. The 2011–12 version contains nine main sections and is nearly 150 pages long. By comparison, the production 'bible' for HBO's drama series *The Wire* was 79 pages (Martin, 2013). The UEFA manual offers an overview of the competition, explaining the 'triangle of mutual benefit'; the relationship between broadcasters, sponsors and football clubs that are 'encircled within the control' of UEFA and TEAM Marketing.

> UEFA controls and conducts the competition and co-ordinates the three partner groups. Additionally, UEFA has appointed TEAM Marketing to secure financial support from the UCL Partners and to facilitate the implementation of the concept on site. (UEFA, 2011:12)

This means UEFA provides sponsorship exposure that is *fully embedded* in the broadcast output and that every Champions League broadcast operation is supervised by TEAM Marketing representatives. UEFA's sponsors for the 2013–14 season included UniCredit, MasterCard, Ford, PlayStation, Gazprom, Heineken, Adidas and HTC. In addition to various credits in and out of commercial breaks during the prescribed coverage, these sponsors often buy additional commercial time in key markets around Champions League broadcasts; in the UK from 2015–16 on BT Sport, previously ITV and Sky Sports. What is the 'triangle of mutual benefit'?

> To ensure the success of the competition everyone must benefit. The Clubs have the opportunity to play on the biggest stage and be financially rewarded for their contribution, whilst the UCL Partners, who provide the competition with worldwide exposure and substantial revenue, benefit from association with an outstanding competition. UEFA/TEAM have pioneered a marketing approach, which ensures that funds raised go directly to the benefit of football. It is also a centralised marketing programme, which also produces clear benefits for Clubs, UCL Partners and spectators. The UCL offers Broadcasters football of the highest quality with the opportunity to broadcast up to 125 UEFA Champions League matches plus 20 play-off matches, providing security of programming to a known calendar. (UEFA, 2011:12)

TEAM Marketing provides supervision ensuring rules are followed and the interests of the partners protected. Conformity is achieved through a combination of:

- Visits to each Club venue.
- Meetings at each venue with the host broadcaster.
- UEFA/TEAM Marketing assigns a coordinating producer to each club for as long as it remains in the tournament.
- The rules and requirements as set out in the Production Manual. (These are explained directly to the host broadcast director by the TEAM producer).
- The host broadcaster is on site for two days for each Matchday (the schedule starts with news requirements on Matchday -1).
- UEFA has a group of quality control (QC) producers that check the final output; this group includes experienced sports directors.

The Manual includes separate detailed guidelines covering:

- Host Broadcast Operations
- TV Graphics
- Venue Operations
- Satellite Distribution
- Content Services

- Information Services
- FAME (Football Administration Management Environment, which handles all requests and bookings).

In terms of coverage UEFA requires that: 'The host broadcaster must use the latest generation of digital equipment on all productions' (UEFA, 2011:19.)

A lot of the information in the manual is technical, from providing copies of unbroken camera-one coverage (the main camera) and of all EVS material. However, two sections focus on editorial matters: section three *Host Broadcast Operations* and section seven, *Content Services*.

Contributors confirm that section seven, *Content Services* includes a wide range of approved content produced and distributed by UEFA to broadcasters, including individual city profiles, numerous Matchday promotional trailers and official graphics elements (titles, logos, backgrounds and animations). On Champions League Matchdays, UEFA provides match-night Highlights, an Instant Highlights feed (available quickly after the games have finished) and further content for mobile and Internet use. Beyond this offer, UEFA also produces a weekly 30-minute UEFA *Champions League Magazine* programme (produced by IMG from the 2012–13 season). There is further access to isolated camera compilations (dramatic angles of match action), plus in-season archive and previous seasons archive. This offer is reminiscent of the approved 'full service' content provided by Premier League Productions for the Premier League.

Host Broadcast Operations, section three, contains what it calls 'principles and match director guidelines' designed to make Champions League coverage as consistent as possible from host broadcaster to host broadcaster:

> The key principle for match directors is to remember they are providing coverage for the multilateral feed so it should be unbiased and aimed at satisfying the viewing preferences of a global audience and not just a specific domestic market. (UEFA, 2011:27)

This is the same guaranteed uniform and stable coverage sought by Formula 1 and the international output of Premier League Productions.

Section three also sets out host broadcast camera positions and the numerous multilateral content production running orders, in other words the editorial content of the multilateral international feed to be offered by each host broadcaster. Typically, a UK broadcaster takes the multi-lateral feed and inserts their own unilateral coverage. The unilateral coverage includes any studio discussion and analysis, pitch-side presentation and interviews. The broadcast output we finally see on television jumps between the multilateral coverage (global) and unilateral injects (local customisation). The reasoning is:

> The multilateral running order (MRO) has been designed to ensure consistency between matches and to inform Broadcasters what coverage to expect during non-playing periods so that they can plan their unilateral productions accordingly. The MRO has been formulated for the following periods: Pre-match, half time, post-match, extra-time and penalties. (UEFA, 2011:44)

All key aspects of Champions League match coverage, from camera placement, replay philosophy, and programme graphics are specified, including minute-by-minute running orders that start at 19.35 (CET) and run through to post-match and to off-air at full-time +6:50 minutes. With as many as eight matches per evening, the Champions League is an impressive logistical operation with all matches kicking off at the same time. Illustrating the extent to which conformity is sought, a reconstructed pre-match multilateral running order (MRO) is set out in table 4.5.

Looking at this indicative running order, an experienced executive producer/director points out:

> As a director, with five minutes to go in a match, I'm sometimes more worried about whether I've put a score caption up at the right time, than whether an incident in the match was a penalty or not. (Executive producer/live sports director, 2013)

Unsurprisingly, UEFA's General Secretary, Gianni Infantino sees issues to do with conformity slightly differently:

> This Production Manual is designed to encourage you to live the UEFA Champions League experience to the full and to help you to provide the best possible coverage for your audience. (UEFA, 2011: Introduction)

In other words, UEFA requires coverage to attain a uniform or approved level. The UEFA Champions League broadcast operation – through the actions of UEFA and TEAM Marketing at each venue and as expressed in the Production Manual – represents a significant level of control exerted

Table 4.5 Reconstructed MRO for UCL Pre-Match

Start (CET)	End (CET)	Dur.	Coverage	Description	Graphics
19.35.00	19.40.00	05.00	Pre-match build up	Teams arrive and walk to dressing rooms players' pitch inspection stadium views fans arriving	
19.40.00	20.10.00	30.00	Pre-multi unilaterals	Multi-camera coverage of Stadium as atmosphere builds Multi-camera coverage of player warm ups	Broadcaster idents
20.10.00	20.14.00	04.00	Warm Ups	Multi-camera coverage of both teams, 15s isolation per player	
20.14.00	20.15.00	01.00	Stadium wide shot		Home team selection Tactical line ups Repeat for away team
20.15.00	20.25.00	10.00	Pre-Multilateral	beauty shot, followed by multi-camera player warm ups	
20.25.00	20.26.00	01.00	Stadium wide shot	Clean shot	Match ID (2m)
20.26.00	20.28.00	02.00	Stadium wide shot		Countdown to TX (2m)
20.28.00	20.30.00	02.00	Stadium wide shot		
20.30.00	20.30.40	00.40	Opening Sequence		Match ID & weather
20.30.40	20.31.00	00.20	Stadium wide shot		
20.31.00	20.31.30	00.30	Stadium atmospher	Crowd home and away shots	
20.31.30	20.34.00	02.30	Key player Isolated shots	Player CUs, super slomo 75s each, home then away Live stadium sounds	

20.34.00	20.35.30	01.30	Stadium wide shot		Home team line up and tactical – 20s each, home then away team
20.35.30	20.36.00	00.30	Stadium wide shot		Home team subs 10s, away team 10s
20.36.00	20.36.30	00.30	Stadium beauty shot	Clean wide shot	
20.36.30	20.37.30	01.00	Star player comparison	Super slomo for each team start player	Player name and stats
20.37.30	20.38.00	00.30	Stadium wide shot		Group standings
20.38.00	20.39.30	01.30	Stadium ambience	Live atmosphere crowd shots, show home and away fans	
20.39.30	20.40.00	00.30	Stadium wide shot		Match ID 20 secs
20.40.00	20.41.00	01.00	Players in tunnel		
20.41.00	20.42.00	01.00	Players walking on pitch		
20.42.00	20.43.15	01.15	Teams line up, UCL Anthem & handshakes		
20.43.15	20.43.40	00.25	Stadium wide shot		Home team line up and tactical
20.43.40	20.44.00	00.20	Coin toss		Officials IDs
20.44.00	20.44.25	00.25	Stadium wide shot		Away team line up and tactical
20.44.25	20.44.50	00.25	Coaches CUs		Coaches name captions
20.44.50	20.45.00	00.10	Main cams shots		
20.45.00			KICK OFF		

Sources: UEFA.com, contributor interviews, author's off-air notes.

by a governing body over the final broadcast output. Whilst broadcasters can provide additional local context, via their unilateral presentation content and channel style, the core match coverage remains firmly in the hands of UEFA because:

> Developments in the commercial and media world have gone hand in hand with football's evolution in recent years. Consequently, UEFA's marketing, commercial and technological activities have intensified considerably. (UEFA, 2009)

Fynn, interviewed in 2003, (Boyle and Haynes, 2004:64) argues that UEFA 'Now recognise through control of sponsorship, advertising and TV rights that they have the power'. This section has demonstrated that this market power goes a very long way to define what the final programmes look and sound like. This is the reality of transformations in sports broadcasting rights.

Conclusion

The continuing migration of market power from broadcasters and media providers upstream to the leagues and federations that control rights was discussed. The changing values and definitions used in sports broadcasting rights were also reviewed.

How increasing levels of control over output have been introduced was illustrated with examples from Formula 1 and the UEFA Champions League. These cases were used to explain how a largely unseen influence is extended to what we, as viewers, finally see and hear on screen.

The chapter opened with a brief review of the nature of intellectual property, including the confusion caused by the *idea/expression dichotomy*. The tendency of copyright to be defined by market-driven principles to demarcate who owns what was also explained. The lack of a homogenised approach to international copyright – and the subsequent reliance on national regulations for enforcement – was noted. An account of the changing values and definitions of sports broadcasting rights highlighted key factors that determine value, before the different ways that rights are broken down (by range, distribution platform, broadcast territory and period of license) were reviewed. Past and present revenues for Premier League broadcasting rights in the UK and overseas were set out.

With the escalating cost of sports broadcasting rights, a corresponding increase in the risks to broadcasters associated with acquiring such rights was noted, including the consequences of over valuing or losing important rights. A broadcaster's perspective on rights was provided, followed by a discussion of the dilemmas that broadcasters face when acquiring expensive sports rights. It was noted that, in the UK, by 2015 only one broadcaster (BSkyB) had a long-term track record in successfully monetising the ownership of expensive Premier League broadcasting rights. With the retention of two packages of Premier League rights for 2016–19 for a relatively modest increase in fees (from £738 million to £960 million) BT is maintaining a strong challenge.

Finally, the important and largely unseen dimension of the prescriptions that are frequently added to broadcasting rights contracts was reviewed. The addition of production prescriptions also indicates a critical division between federation-approved international *coverage* and the localised *presentation* (content structured *around* sports events) that is now provided by rights holding broadcasters and media suppliers. Whilst providing access to large audiences, broadcasters' influence of actual event coverage is becoming more marginal. Despite a scarcity of academic scrutiny this is a very important development that illustrates a 'quiet accretion of restrictions' through the application of IP rights (Drahos and Braithwaite, 2002:4).

The battle to acquire the most appealing sports broadcasting rights has intensified in response to the rising tide of commercialism in UK sports and the continued marketisation of broadcasting. In the same way that broadcasting rights can be considered to follow one cycle behind developments in technology – usually three years – then regulators in the EU and UK can be seen to follow another step behind broadcasting rights. How, among other things, regulators tackle market power and market failure in sports television is discussed in Chapter 5.

5
Regulation

Regulation is the third pre-production factor that influences what television sport we can see, including where and when we can see it. As Evens, Iosifidis and Smith (2013) summarise, since the 1990s:

> ... the UK sports broadcasting market has been subject to almost constant scrutiny by a whole series of (UK and EU) policymakers and regulatory authorities. Broadly speaking, attention has focussed on two key areas: first, legislation designed to ensure that coverage of major national sporting events remains available to all television viewers – listed events legislation: and secondly, the application of competition law to the sports broadcasting market in an effort to reduce the market power of the dominant pay-TV broadcaster, BSkyB. (Evens, Iosifidis and Smith, 2013:203)

This chapter examines how different levels of intervention impact on sports television; several associated but less talked about dimensions include content regulation, regional and independent production quotas and the impact of Transfer of Undertakings Regulations (TUPE).

When it comes to regulation, my experience of sports producers is that they often prefer a slightly standoff approach to many issues, particularly Transfer of Undertakings (TUPE), hence they do not always communicate a fully formed view (in the same way a miner may know a lot about extracting coal but, perhaps, a bit less about the coal mining industry). It is fair to say that broadcasters and executives from independent sports production companies tend to have more direct contact with regulatory and competition outcomes.

Why has television sport attracted so much attention from UK and EU policymakers and regulatory authorities? With UK sports becoming more commercially oriented and with the marketisation of broadcasting, numerous long-established social and cultural values have been put aside in favour of 'the financialisation of everything' (Harvey, 2005:33). Consequently, sport and broadcasting are now globally distributed and privatised goods. Boyle and Haynes (2004:52) write, a 're-regulation of broadcasting is taking place within a more commercial and market-driven frame of reference'. This process has been intensified by developments in digital technology. Typically, leagues and pay-TV providers often call for a free market approach with less regulation, while political economists advocate a more rigorous application of competition law together with listed event regulation. Whilst sympathising with the political economy position, discussions seldom foreground the *full range* of regulatory measures that apply to television sports production – some of which can determine *where* a production is made (regional production quotas) and *who* can work on it (Transfer of Undertakings – TUPE – that applies when a production contract moves from one company to another). This chapter redresses the balance.

Boyle and Haynes (2004:163) raise an interesting point: 'football has always worn its civic responsibility lightly'. As football rewrites its cultural contract with fans 'primarily along commercial lines protected under the sign of the law' (Boyle and Haynes, 2004:79), the cultural, social and historical aspects of many clubs have been commodified and turned into elements of global branding strategy. We end up with a commercially driven Premier League operating within a wider economic climate in which the market remains the central driver. In such conditions fans of Hull City protest about a name change to Hull Tigers and Cardiff City fans object to their team changing their traditional blue shirts for red, as red is considered a 'lucky' colour in Asia. Commercial conditions produce a league that is very different from the more inclusive structure adopted by the Bundesliga in 2002 and where football is considered a *public good* and activities, including club ownership, are grounded in the local community. In contrast to the market-driven Premier League, the Bundesliga took the view that football is one of the last activities that really brings people together, so ticket prices are set to ensure a wide range of fans can attend. Finding a balance between commerce and culture, market principles and wider social meaning, is the daunting challenge for regulators. Intervention by media regulators and competition authorities appears to be the only limitation currently placed on the conduct of leagues and federations.

The sheer pace at which technology (including new methods and means of delivery) and sports broadcasting rights have developed since the early 1990s, has posed serious problems for regulators and policy-makers. As Boyle and Haynes (2004:165) summarise: 'regulators strive to keep pace with a digital mediascape which threatens to perpetually run ahead of regulatory frameworks'. The recent move by federations to take control of their own host broadcast operations and global content distribution could leave regulators even further adrift.

So far this book has considered ways that television sport in the UK has adopted more overtly commercial models typically found in the US, but when it comes to broadcasting policy and regulation very different values are in play, as Jeanrenaud and Kesenne (2006:6) explain:

> In the US sport is seen as a commodity which has to be redesigned as viewers' preferences or sponsors' requirements change. In Europe, by contrast, sport is considered part of the cultural heritage. The dominant position in Europe is that sport cannot be reduced to being merely an audience-generating mechanism and that there is a need to preserve both its identity and independence. (European Commission, 1999)

Still considering the wider picture, Smith (2009) highlights the growth of the regulatory state as part of a general shift from government to governance associated with the withdrawal of the state from many activities as part of neoliberal thinking. Whilst facilitating conditions conducive to a free market is an objective, monopolistic tendencies still need to be curbed. Therefore a central concern of regulation is the control of market power. Given that broadcasting is an oligopolistic market, then strategic behaviour, such as first mover strategy often adopted by BSkyB, can offer advantages. On the other hand, in a market with only a small number of players, a dominant position, like that held by BSkyB, also risks infringing the rules. Controlling market power in sports broadcasting in the UK and Europe is a recurring theme.

It was the deregulation of broadcasting policy associated with the landmark 1990 Broadcasting Act that provided significant momentum for the transformation of television sport in the UK, including the arrival of direct competition to the established terrestrial networks from satellite broadcasters; the previously closed world of broadcasting was to be exposed to the rigours of the free market. The 1990 Act also included the first formal quota for independent productions. Doyle (2002:161) reminds us that government policy initiative and regulatory measures strongly influence the economic performances of media markets while Evens, Iosifidis and Smith (2013) see too much emphasis on preserving the investments of pay-TV operators. The influence of

EU-level media regulation and competition authorities on policymaking and UK broadcasters is also noted by Smith (2009). Scrutiny is applied to both the demand side (the ways that broadcasting rights are sold upstream by leagues and federations) and the supply side, the market in which the final programmes are aired. However, it is argued here that the discussion would benefit from being widened to include the activities of:

- Leagues and federations (principally those that issue broadcasting rights).
- Broadcasters and media providers (buyers of broadcasting rights and owners of distribution platforms).
- Broadcasters, production companies and producers that provide the finished content.

5.1 The list of protected events

Speaking on 21 July 2010, the then Sports Minister Hugh Robertson (Conservative) supported the principle of protecting major sports events for free-to-air coverage. The two-tiered list of protected events continues to apply in late 2015.

As early as the 1930s, during the years of BBC monopoly, an annual calendar of broadcast events had been created, one that resonated with the winter and summer seasons of sport in the UK (Scannell and Cardiff, 1991). Delivering important sporting events to a national audience became a cornerstone of the BBC's PSB remit (Boyle and Haynes, 2000:69). Arguing that it was promoting events to a national audience, the BBC resisted paying sports broadcasting rights fees. In the 1950s the removal of the BBC's monopoly status, as the Conservative government planned to introduce commercial television via the Television Act of 1954, raised concerns over bidding wars for broadcasting rights, Smith (2009) provides a good account. The arrival of ITV saw the BBC and Parliament claim that 'wealthy commercial interests might outbid the BBC and ... deprive the BBC of events they expected to see on the national service' (Sendall, 1982:52). The BBC proposed the government draw up a list of national events which could not be broadcast on an exclusive basis by any broadcaster, thus averting bidding wars for broadcasting rights. The list of protected rights was first set out in the Television Act of 1954 although this was, essentially, a gentleman's agreement (Barnett, 1990).

The spectre of bidding wars was raised again in the 1980s and the list of protected events was redrafted as part of the Cable and Broadcasting

Act 1984 (Smith, 2009:9) and by 1985 the protected list of national events had become statutory. The general commercialisation of broadcasting under the Conservative government continued during the 1980s and 1990s as policy restrictions were gradually watered down; the landmark 1990 Broadcasting Act replaced the 1984 Act. Opponents of the 1990 Act claimed that it was enabling an unwelcome Americanisation of British broadcasting. With new legislation the Independent Broadcast Authority (IBA) was replaced by the Independent Television Commission (ITC), a light-touch regulator that was, in turn, replaced in December 2003 by the super-regulator Ofcom.

The arrival of BSkyB in 1990 and its subsequent acquisition, not only of the Premier League broadcasting rights, but also of rights to the Football League, England's home matches and golf's Ryder Cup established a 'virtuous circle of more subscribers/more sports rights' (Booth and Doyle, 1997:280). In turn, this prompted debate about whether sport was a *public good* or a *private good*; was it right that the nation's favourite game be hidden behind a pay wall? More than 20 years later, an interesting parallel can be drawn between the commercial trajectory of the Premier League and the Bundesliga, where the German league understood the wider social value of football as a *public good*. The Bundesliga maintains a 50+1 ownership rule, ensuring clubs are (a) grounded in the local community (and not owned by wealthy foreign investors), and (b) are fully focussed on football not financial activities. Access for all levels of society is ensured through affordable admission prices offered at Bundesliga grounds.

Returning to the UK, in 1995 a situation had arisen, argued dissenters, where three quarters of the nation would be excluded from major sports leaving access only for those wealthy enough to subscribe. The 1990 Broadcasting Act's restriction on the pay-per-view broadcasting of listed events was extended to include subscription broadcasting, a return to the position set out in the 1984 Cable and Broadcasting Act. This is an example of how the pace of transformation in technology and in broadcasting rights had started to outstrip the regulators' ability to react.

By 1997 the Department of Culture, Media and Sport (DCMS) introduced the idea that a sport on the list of protected events must have a *special national resonance*, an event that unites the nation and is a shared point on the national calendar. Not all sports actually wanted protected status and sought, instead, to negotiate the most lucrative commercial deals available, usually with BSkyB as with the English Cricket Board (ECB) in 2009 when it opposed inclusion on the list as it would reduce the economic value it could achieve for broadcasting rights in a free market. To some sports authorities revenue from rights was more important than being seen by larger numbers of viewers on terrestrial television. BSkyB has frequently called upon leagues and federations for support following challenges from regulators and competition authorities.

Unlike the UK, there is no list of protected events in the US. The US Major Leagues have managed to maintain a strong presence on the four commercial free-to-air networks and have not migrated wholesale to pay-TV as the Premier League has done in the UK. In another major difference, the US Sport Broadcasting Act of 1961 exempted the collective selling of sponsored telecasting, or cartel behaviour, from anti-trust legislation as authorities accepted the need for a governance structure in sport, including horizontal arrangements aimed at enhancing competitive balance within each league (Fort, 2006:429). The Telecommunications Act of 1996 went on to remove most price regulations and the main frame of reference is the Sherman Antitrust Act. But the conduct of the leagues themselves includes an important difference insofar as they have adopted rules that, ultimately, maintain the value of their broadcasting rights. The three broad regulatory principles adopted by the leagues include, (a) a fair (equal) share of television rights to all member clubs, (b) salary caps for club rosters (including named franchise players), and (c) a reverse-order-of finish draft system for players entering the league (Desbordes, 2006). Evens, Iosifidis and Smith (2013) argue that the US case:

> ...illustrates that increased exposure and higher audience ratings via free-to-air television can serve the interest of teams, leagues, broadcasters, advertisers, sponsors and viewers alike. (Evens, Iosifidis and Smith, 2013:228)

Whilst professional sports have always been more malleable in the US – particularly when accommodating the demands of television – it does not follow that the country has foregone all sporting cultural heritage. Finding a balance, between commercial concerns and wider social and cultural benefits, is a key issue in the UK and Europe.

Concern that the market for the most appealing sports broadcasting rights was becoming dominated by commercial players – the Kirch Group in Germany, Canal Plus in France and BSkyB in the UK – led the EU to adopt the UK's approach of providing a protected list of sports events via legislation. Evens, Smith and Iosifidis (2013) explain how the European Parliament (EP) used a review of the Television Without

Frontiers Directive (TVWF) as a convenient means to press for EU-wide legislation. In November 1996, the EP approved an amendment to the TVWF Directive to ensure that coverage of sporting events of general interest are available on free-to-air TV (EC, 1997). In February 1997, an EU system of listed events based on the principle of mutual recognition was articulated; no broadcaster would be allowed to circumvent the rules governing protected events in any other EU state. Major event legislation was formally adopted as part of the renewed 1997 TVWF Directive and subsequently incorporated into the 2007 Audiovisual Media Service Directive (Evens, Iosifidis and Smith, 2013:77). The Davis Committee (2009) was set up to review the UK's protected list of events and recommended a return to a single list of protected events. Further decisions were deferred leaving the current list of category A and category B events, as published by the DCMS, intact. Category A includes full live event coverage whilst category B provides for secondary coverage (primarily same day highlights shown on the terrestrial networks):

Table 5.1   Protected List of Events (Groups A and B)

Category A Events – Full live coverage protected
The Olympic Games
FIFA World Cup Finals
European Championships Finals
FA Cup Final
Scottish FA Cup Final
The Grand National
The Derby
Wimbledon Lawn Tennis Finals
Rugby League Challenge Cup Final
Rugby Union World Cup Final

Category B Events – Secondary coverage protected
England Home Test Cricket Matches
Non-Finals Play at Wimbledon
All other matches at the Rugby World Cup Finals
6 Nations Rugby Tournament matches involving home countries
The Commonwealth Games
IAAF World Athletics Championships
The Cricket World Cup – finals, semifinals and matches featuring
    home nation's teams
The Ryder Cup
The Open Golf Championship

Source: DCMS.

Without the list of protected events it is hard to see how the publicly funded BBC would have a meaningful foothold on top tier sports broadcasting rights and, even so, two of the most popular football competitions, the Premier League and the UEFA Champions League, are not included on either list. Given their exclusion from the lists, perhaps it is no surprise that the activities of Premier League and UEFA should prove of particular interest to regulators and competition authorities in the UK and Europe?

5.2 The Premier League

The Office of Fair Trading (OFT) referred the Premier League's exclusive rights deals of 1992 and 1996 to the Restrictive Practices Court (RPC), where the OFT claimed that the collective selling of all Premier League clubs' television rights by the Premier League was illegal (Boyle and Haynes, 2004). However, the business of team sports is no ordinary business. For Neale (1964:14): 'It is clear that professional sports are a natural monopoly, marked by definite peculiarities both in the structure and in the functioning of their markets'. Leagues are necessary to professional sport; a single team cannot supply the entire market because it would have no other team to play. However, a single league can supply the entire market in conditions of a natural monopoly (Dobson and Goddard, 2007:5). It is also the case that competition between different sports is more likely than competition between rival leagues within the same sport; the Premier League is a rare example of a new league successfully replacing the dominant incumbent league (Fort, 2006:150). In professional sport, many basic economic rules are inverted – Neale (1964) highlights the *single-entity* action by leagues leading to profitable economic outcomes, naming it 'the peculiar economics of team sports'. Finally, leagues are necessary to provide competition and uncertainty of outcome, in addition to scheduling matches, providing officials and other joint venture conduct. There is an argument to be made that the confusion between the need for sporting competition and sporting monopoly – accepted in the US – has never been fully resolved in the UK and Europe. In part this is due to the cultural value placed on sport in the UK and Europe. To some extent this reaction is reminiscent of the reluctance to embrace professionalism (over amateurism) in the UK in the 1960s. The transformation of professional sport suggests a revision of what we, in the UK and Europe, expect from elite professional sport would be useful. It is worth repeating that it is within the gift of leagues and federations to turn their focus away from purely commercial outcomes, as demonstrated by the Bundesliga.

In July 1999, the Restrictive Practices Court ruled that the Premier League's deals with BSkyB did not impose unreasonable restrictions on the clubs, nor was the agreement contrary to the public interest (Gratton and Solberg, 2007:159). In defending its position BSkyB argued that it was legitimate for a single broadcaster to retain exclusive broadcasting rights for a limited time, as long as rights were regularly renegotiated and sold in a fair and open manner (Boyle and Haynes, 2004: Haynes, 2005). From 2001, we see Premier League rights being sold every three years whereas, previously, they had been sold in five year (1992–97) and four year (1997–2001) periods.

In 2000, the Premier League started to unbundle the various broadcasting rights it was offering for auction. Three packages were subsequently created (a) to reduce the risk of further intervention from the competition authorities and (b) to increase Premier League revenues. For the 2001–04 period, BSkyB secured 106 games and NTL withdrew its bid due to financial problems. ITV secured the rights to highlights, leaving the BBC with no Premier League football at all (no Premier League match has, so far, been broadcast live on free-to-air television in the UK).

In December 2002, the Competition Directorate of the European Commission launched its own investigation into the selling of Premier League broadcasting rights (Haynes, 2005:75). According to Smith (2009) the Commission set out to negate the potential anti-competitive effects from the collective selling of Premier League broadcasting rights. Boyle and Haynes (2004) add:

> The key to the whole negotiation and bidding process was the EC investigation and its 'guiding hand' in the structure of the deal. While not prescriptive, the EC edict that collective selling could only exist where the consumer ultimately benefitted from wider choice and no broadcaster could exclusively sew up all the rights clearly influenced the initial tender document issued by the Premier League in June 2003. (Boyle and Haynes, 2004:47.)

Initially, the rights for the period 2004–07 consisted of a gold package of 38 matches starting at 16.00 on Sunday afternoon, a silver package of 38 matches on Monday evenings, midweek and Sundays at 14.00, and a bronze package of 92 matches on Saturdays at 13.00 and 17.15 – a total of 138 matches, up from the previous total of 106. However, after the initial bidding process had begun, the Premier League separated the bronze package into two licenses, creating, in all, four packages of live rights. Boyle and Haynes (2004) point out a traditional highlights package was available, plus a new package of rights that allowed a broadcaster or a club channel to screen 'as live' re-runs from midnight on match day. Additionally, short-form clip rights to all 380 Premier League matches were available for distribution on mobile phones from five minutes after the end of the games. It appeared that the attention of regulators and competition authorities was having some impact. Or was it? In August 2003, BSkyB successfully bid for all four live match packages giving them more games for less money when compared to the deal for 2001–04 (Boyle and Haynes, 2004:49). It is doubtful that strengthening BSkyB's position was the preferred outcome of this intervention.

Under further pressure from the Competition Commission, the Premier League agreed that BSkyB should sublicense eight matches per season to another broadcaster in an auction process. Haynes (2005:75) reports that BSkyB executives saw the leakage of eight games as undermining the exclusivity of the rights they had just purchased. However, a reserve price for the rights was agreed and, as no broadcaster met this price, the eight sublicensed matches reverted to BSkyB.

But there had been concessions; the period for rights was reduced to three years (Haynes, 2005:76) and the Premier League was required to ensure there was a second broadcaster that held live rights for the period 2007–10 (Gratton and Solberg, 2007:6). In 2005, it was agreed that live rights would be sold in six balanced packages (of 23 matches) with no one bidder being able to buy all six packages. The door was finally opened to a new broadcaster. BSkyB secured four packages and 92 matches, whilst newcomer Setanta acquired two packages, totalling 46 matches. Whilst the European Commission had successfully ended BSkyB's monopoly of live rights to Premier League football it is questionable whether 'the consumer benefitted from wider choice' – yes, there was more choice available but viewers that wanted to see all Premier League matches now had to buy two subscriptions at greater cost. With no live rights available to free-to-air broadcasters, it could be argued that it was not in the best interests of consumers. Increased competition for rights *did* result in an escalation in the prices paid to the Premier League, a very favourable outcome.

In the next rights issue (2010–13) Setanta was not able to match its previous bid price (Sweney, 2009). However, the company was able to secure a single package of rights for a reduced outlay, due to the restriction placed on the Premier League to ensure that rights were split between two broadcasters. The loss of a package (from two packages including 46 games, down to one with 23 games) raised questions about Setanta's strategic position in the UK pay-TV market. Failing to attract sufficient new subscribers, the company struggled to pay the fees due to the Premier League and, in summer 2009, fell into administration (Smith, 2009:17). The rights were quickly re-auctioned and awarded to ESPN (Robinson, 2009).

In 2012, working for IMG (the producer of Premier League Productions), predictions about a new bidder for Premier League rights occupied industry insiders, with Al Jazeera expected to fulfil this role. However, it was BT Sport that emerged and, by providing some serious financial competition to BSkyB, helped to propel domestic revenue for the period 2013–16 to an all-time high in excess of £3 billion for the seven packages of live matches offered (Press Association, 2012). The winner, once again, was the Premier League. Former BSkyB Head of programming David Elstein added his view that BSkyB:

> ... is also an extremely tough competitor, and treats regulators with as little regard as it treats commercial rivals. More than 20 years ago, its mantra was: we will strangle cable before cable strangles us. It has taken on the likes of the Office of Fair Trading, the Competition Commission and the broadcasting regulator, Ofcom, as each of them has tried to level up the playing field in television. (Elstein, 2010)

Have the regulators succeeded in levelling the playing field? In 2014 BSkyB's hold on Premier League football remained robust. As in previous cases, viewers wishing to see all available Premier League matches are required to pay for two subscriptions for 2013–16, one for Sky Sports and another for BT Sport (in late 2015, existing BT broadband customers still receive basic BT Sport for free). Had even one package of live rights ended up being available on a free-to-air broadcaster then it would be easier to see the point of this intervention – a split between two pay-TV services delivers less benefit than providing wider access via free-to-air broadcast. This underlines the difficulties of regulators and competition authorities in keeping up with the activities of the Premier League, BSkyB and BT Sport. Whilst the application of legislation via the list of protected events offers tangible results, the results when applying competition law in respect of the Premier League appears harder to justify.

5.3   The UEFA Champions League

The premier European club competition was re-launched in 1992 as the UEFA Champions League (UCL), with the new format replacing the

European Champion's Cup. Unlike the Premier League, coverage of the UEFA Champions League took much longer to migrate to pay-TV in the UK than it did in many other countries across Europe where it had already found a home. So, whilst BSkyB was able to show exclusive live Premier League matches from 1992–93, it was not until 2003 that the UCL first appeared on BSkyB. BSkyB paid approximately £240 million, while ITV paid £160 million giving the free-to-air broadcaster first picks of Tuesday night fixtures (van Wijk, 2013).

The split-broadcasting arrangement, somewhat like the Premier League but, crucially, including a free-to-air outlet, was due to intervention from the European Competition Commission as it sought to investigate the selling of football rights in a range of media markets across Europe. Whilst the Commission accepted the declaration of the specific characteristics of sport adopted by the European Council at Nice in 1999, the EU, according to Boyle and Haynes (2004), increasingly viewed sport as a business, particularly point 15 that recognised the sale of broadcasting rights is one of the primary sources of income for certain sports (EC, 1999). The EC investigation into the anti-competitive joint selling of Champions League rights resulted in no single national broadcaster being able to acquire sole live rights to the competition from 2003–04 (Haynes, 2005:66). With 14 categories of rights being marketed centrally by UEFA and TEAM Marketing, new rights were created which meant that more broadcasters might be able to secure rights. This allowed BSkyB to acquire the majority of rights in the UK, reducing ITV's eventual broadcast output to a single match-night per round of games.

According to Boyle and Haynes (2004), at this time a number of rights reverted back to individual clubs and there was a greater emphasis on mobile and Internet rights, with UEFA seeking to grow revenue alongside an expanding European broadband market. It remains unclear to what extent this market has materialised, as television coverage remains by far the most popular medium through which to view Champions League content. In terms of additional competition to acquire Champions League rights from 2015–18, then BT chief executive Gavin Patterson made good on his promise that BT Sport would bid for these rights (van Wijk, 2013). In November 2013, BT was granted exclusive rights to broadcast 350 Champions League and Europa League matches a season for 3 years at a cost of £897 million (Calvin, 2013). Although Goodley and Monaghan (2013) report Patterson as claiming to 'give sport back to the fans', and acknowledging that BT had injected 'a welcome element of competition' into the market, it remains to be seen how this rights acquisition sits (a) with the requirement that rights should not be held by a single broadcaster, and (b) how BT plans to make some matches available free-to-air. BT's channel positions on Freeview, the free-to-air digital terrestrial television service, are the most likely platform to make these games available from 2015–16.

Given the rights sale to BT Sport the benefits of EU-wide intervention in the auctioning of Champions League broadcasting rights could be contested. However, of potentially even greater significance is UEFA's own introduction of the *Financial Fair Play Regulations* (FFP), first approved in 2010. According to UEFA's website these rules are set out to:

- Introduce more discipline and rationality in club football finances.
- Decrease pressure on salaries and transfer fees and limit inflationary effect.
- Encourage clubs to compete within their revenues.
- Encourage long-term investments in the youth sector and infrastructure.
- Protect the long-term viability of European club football.
- Ensure clubs settle their liabilities on a timely basis.

The FFP regulations came into full effect for the 2013–14 season. Whilst FFP is not the completely business-oriented closed system used in US leagues, it is the strongest suggestion yet that regulations similar in intention to those adopted by US leagues, including salary caps and other agreed measures, including the reverse order-of-finish player draft system and naming of franchise players, designed to promote competitive balance and uncertainty of outcome (critical to maintaining the value of broadcasting rights) are being considered for application in a European context. In May 2014 UEFA sanctioned Premier League club Manchester City under the Financial Fair Play Regulations imposing a fine of £50 million and restrictions on their Champions League squad for the 2014–15 season (Gibson, 2014). UEFA sanctioned nine clubs that breached FFP rules.

The argument here does not seek to devalue the wider benefits from listed event regulation and the application of competition law, but, in addition to these measures, the leagues and federations should be encouraged to take more responsibility for balancing their books and for managing their affairs more constructively, including broadcasting activities and wider social outcomes. This path is likely to be more beneficial to more people in the longer term. Both the German Bundesliga and UEFA have demonstrated ways to engage with their civic responsibility; the Premier League might also consider this approach.

5.4 Ofcom, UK market regulation

As a result of the Communications Act 2003 regulatory powers in the UK passed from the ITC to the newly formed Ofcom. Ofcom's duties include:

- Managing, regulating and assignment of the electromagnetic spectrum and licensing portions of the spectrum for television broadcasting.
- Specifying the Broadcast Code, including mandatory rules including the protection of children, harm and offense, crime, religion, impartiality and accuracy, elections, fairness, privacy, sponsorship and commercial references.
- Rules on the amount and distribution of advertising.
- Undertaking public consultations.
- Dealing with viewer complaints.

Ofcom has also developed Terms of Trade/Codes of Practice that apply to rights deals between independent producers and commissioners/broadcasters. These terms were introduced in the Communications Act 2003, with independent producers retaining a share of IP rights on created content (particularly secondary rights). In sport, secondary rights are retained by the leagues and federations and sold as 'overseas' rights.

Returning to questions of market power and the supply of programmes in the downstream market, such investigations are not limited to the EU Competition Commission. Between 2007 and 2010, Ofcom completed a review of the pay-TV market in the UK (Ofcom, 2010). The review followed complaints from BT, Virgin Media, Top-Up TV and Setanta that BSkyB exerted a vicious circle of control that crushes competition (Smith, 2009:20). In particular, it was the ability of BSkyB to determine carriage charges – both for rival channels on its own platform (and for EPG access) and for carrying its own brands, such as Sky Sports – that was considered problematic. The outcome required BSkyB to lower the wholesale prices it charged the rival companies for Sky Sports 1 and Sky Sports 2. Ofcom appears exasperated by the experience as expressed in the Pay TV Statement (para:1.25):

> Our review of these negotiations reveals lengthy and ultimately fruitless discussions over a number of years between Sky and other pay-TV operators over possible wholesale of Sky's premium channels. This impasse has remained despite, as Sky agrees, there being an

immediate financial benefit to Sky from wholesale supply. We believe this is because Sky is acting on two strategic incentives – to protect its retail business on its own satellite platform, and to reduce the risk of stronger competition for content rights. (Ofcom, 2010:7)

Former BSkyB executive David Elstein adds his view: 'BSkyB has become notorious for taking on regulators, winning some battles, prolonging others, and generally giving the competition authorities pause before embarking on any restraining course'. (Elstein, 2010)

What does this constant skirmishing mean? Is regulation pointless? Have broadcasters like BSkyB and organisations like the Premier League and UEFA become too powerful? The argument is that the more powerful the league or broadcaster is then the more necessary potential intervention becomes, particularly where there is monopoly provision. Smith (2009:22) concludes that the role played by the EU *has* enhanced the capacity of the UK government to pursue its desired outcomes. My own view is, whilst regulatory principles are to be applauded in their intention, the actual outcomes, at least in the cases cited above, leave a lot to be desired.

In the case of Ofcom's Pay TV review, in August 2012 the Competition Appeals Tribunal (CAT) said that Ofcom's entire case against BSkyB was unfounded (Hewlett, 2012), although, on 26 April 2014 BT was granted the right to appeal (BSkyB, 2013:13). While Ofcom was less successful in limiting BSkyB's activities, in 2012 BT announced its arrival as a very well-funded rival to BSkyB in the competitive market to acquire appealing sports rights. In 2014 Ofcom announced a new review into whether BSkyB should still have to wholesale its key sports channels given changes in the market (Mance, 2014).

Whilst this is a challenging area, in my view some of the attention regulators and competition authorities that have focused on sports broadcasting often appear (a) to be too late (regulating on technology and broadcasting rights that have had a chance to become well-established as practice is usually problematic), and (b) often seems to misunderstand some of the 'peculiar economics of professional sports' (Neale, 1964). The situation is symptomatic of powerful and extremely well-funded leagues and pay-TV providers using technology and rights to serve their own commercial interests first and foremost. However, it seems reasonable to ask if more lasting solutions might be found by considering the experience of the US leagues and in self-motivated league and federation action, including improved governance and increased civic responsibility as was the case with the re-launch of the German Bundesliga in 2002. As the Premier League continues to expand its own content production arm, including a 24/7 Premier League global channel, and federations provide international host broadcasting services for their own events it is unclear how and where regulators will be able to intervene in the future.

5.5 Regulating content production

Discussion of regulation and intervention tends to be focused on upstream activities and seldom considers the direct contact with broadcasters and producers that regularly occurs downstream on the content supply side. For example, each Ofcom license requires all broadcasters (and therefore all producers, whether in-house or independent) to comply with the Broadcasting Code on content standards (Ofcom, 2013). This interaction is worth noting.

For sports broadcasting, the content standards categories that apply have become more extensive with the corresponding expansion of sports output over the past 20 years. These include: the protection of children, harm and offense, crime, religion, impartiality and accuracy, elections, fairness, privacy, sponsorship and commercial references. Of these, probably only elections and, perhaps, crime are less relevant, although an increasing number of betting scandals and, in 2015, the FBI's investigation into the conduct of FIFA suggest no assumptions can be made.

Among many active sports producers the Broadcasting Code is simply not well known; the level of operational knowledge is, in my direct experience over the last decade, very low. As a senior executive producer for a leading independent confirms:

> Young producers are not aware of regulations like fairness and privacy. We did our stints as assistant producers and didn't become full producers until we were ready to do so. Too many young sports producers are promoted quickly and are not aware of their responsibilities. (Senior executive, Independent production, 2013)

As making sure producers *do* know their responsibility seems a reasonable expectation this raises a question about why these responsibilities are not always well known. A senior producer explains a difference unique to television sport: the apparent hegemony found in sports production culture. This is a kind of self-policing of accepted practice that represents a form of covert compliance in itself:

> Most people [sports producers] grew up watching sport so, when they become producers, they tend to replicate what they saw and what they think is appropriate. It's a closed world. You can't step out of the box. (Senior sports producer, independent sports production, 2012)

Tunstall (1993:2) argued that television sport was a closed world. More than 20 years later it appears that not much has changed. Television sport relies on producers behaving predictably within unspoken but consensual parameters. Consequently, when it comes to the Broadcasting Code there is, in my direct experience, very little in the way of training for independent sports producers. Guidance, when it is available, tends to come from the commissioning channel, whether it is the robust position taken by BSkyB in following Ofcom rules, through to an extremely relaxed position like that of Trace Sports. In other words, the frame of reference can be rather wide.

Typical examples that attract the attention of compliance officers include the increasing commercialisation of top sports stars, particularly around sponsorship, branded clothing and equipment, so undue prominence can be a problematic area. Whilst Formula 1 presents so many sponsors logos that none may stand out, Sir Alex Ferguson can, in October 2013, gain blanket coverage across numerous broadcasts promoting his new book. Even apparently innocent mistakes, like a misplaced shot of a player tying up a branded football boot prior to training (shown, say, in a short feature) can fall foul of the rules and will need to be re-edited at the production company's expense.

For sports events that heavily feature betting, for example Channel Four's horse-racing, a balance is required in the prominence given to, say, Littlewoods betting options over services from other providers.

Harm and offence is not limited to more obvious shots of players mouthing obscenities on screen (or of foul language or racist abuse being chanted in the ground), In late October 2013, BT Sport fell foul, for a second time in just 24 hours, of crude and offensive gestures that were made by in-vision guests during two different football shows (Sale, 2013).

Between January 2011 and July 2012 I produced 140 x 26 minute documentaries for IMG on behalf of Trace Sports. In these films I dealt with issues of privacy – from revealing where a person lived, to showing the license plate on their car – in the great majority of the films.

Privacy cropped up the most, with undue prominence and other commercial issues (such as sponsorship) cropping up in many. In a period where constant access to Internet and YouTube content is taken for granted, inexperienced sports producers appear to be less aware of the Broadcasting Code. And this lack of understanding can even extend to broadcasters. A revealing example is found with Trace Sports as it constantly pushed IMG for access to top football players. Suggesting ways to improve access, a senior Trace Sports executive attended a private party given by Didier Drogba (at the time playing for Chelsea FC). Speaking in 2012, the executive confirmed that she had covertly recorded material from Drogba's event (using a mobile phone), posted it on YouTube, badged as Trace Sport content, and had a very large number of hits. The Trace executive did not accept this conduct infringed Ofcom privacy laws even though the material was covertly recorded and broadcast without permission.

Whilst it is easy to argue that values, such as the Broadcasting Code, need to be supported and upheld across the downstream supply side, it is apparent that emerging digital platforms, user-driven content and federation-based productions will increasingly challenge such values and how they are implemented. That a major media provider like BT Sport can fall outside these guidelines is another reason for concern.

5.6   Regional and independent production quotas

The largest impact of regulation on sports broadcasting in the UK is found in regional production quotas. Senior independent sports production executives have described this impact as 'massive'. Regional quotas are frequently paired with independent production quotas, allowing broadcasters that outsource content to complete two quota requirements with a single commission.

Historically, the independent production sector has delivered high levels of content for PSBs. The creation of Channel Four as a publisher-broadcasters and the formal introduction, through the 1990 Broadcasting Act, of a statutory 25% independent quota for the BBC were important drivers in developing the UK's independent production economy (HMSO, 1990).

Again, the thinking behind such quotas is rational, well-intended and hard to argue with. However, the reality on the production supply side is very often at odds with the objectives. As an executive producer at an independent that regularly supplies material to the BBC said in 2013: 'The BBC has to do a certain amount of regional and independent

production hours, so it decides to place its snooker production outside'.
In this case outside is an independent and regional production company
based in Scotland. The executive producer continues:

> The rules state that 75% of the production must be generated from
> that region. Unfortunately, there are not the outside broadcast com-
> panies in Scotland, let alone the experienced snooker producers,
> directors, assistant producers, cameramen and others to get any-
> where near this figure. It is a complete farce. (Executive producer,
> independent production, 2013)

The company in question has a single representative based in Glasgow
with the senior staff based in London spending a great deal of time
wondering who and how this production can meet the qualifying
regulations.

From my own experience working in the independent sector I am
aware of other examples. Channel Four's *Football Italia* was chosen to
fulfill the broadcasters' regional production quota. As a result, the production moved from London to Yorkshire (Sheffield, then Leeds), cities
that do not offer direct flights to Italy where the programme was shot.
In this case, a proportion of the staff *was* regionally based, but more
came from the north west of England than from Yorkshire. The production was supervised and funded from London. Some sports productions
do sit more comfortably within regional production quotas, particularly
where an event may be based in that region, for example some BBC darts
coverage.

The trend towards increasing specialisation in sports productions,
combined with limited contracts (limited in budget and in duration)
threatens to undermine the intentions of such regulation; it can become
a box-ticking operation by broadcasters. Speaking to a range of contributors, including several senior executives, it is apparent that, in a number
of cases, a degree of obfuscation is involved in meeting all the conditions required under these quotas. Therefore, the extent to which the
quotas help regional development might be questioned.

5.7   Transfer of Undertakings Regulations (TUPE)

While broadcasters and media providers respond to upstream tender
processes that allocate sports broadcasting rights, an important part of
the downstream supply side production economy involves subsequent

tender documents called Requests for Production (RFP) or Invitation to Tender (ITT). These tenders are issued by rights-holding broadcasters, media providers and federations and are concerned with a range of outputs, from a single sports production for a federation right through to a broadcaster's entire sports output, as was the case for ITV Sport in 2009 and for a large proportion of BT Sports production in 2012. The respondents are mostly independent sports production companies, for example IMG Sports Media, Sunset + Vine, North One TV (formerly Chrysalis), Endemol Sport and Century TV, as they compete to win these contracts and build their businesses using a cost plus percentage fee model that, typically, delivers small and sometimes even negligible profit margins.

The UK has implemented the EC's Acquired Rights Directive 1981 amended in 1998 and replaced in 2006 with new regulations (Keter and Jarrett, 2011), on *Transfer of Undertakings (Protection of Employment) Regulations 2006* or TUPE. The regulations are designed to protect employees whose business is being transferred to another business – employee's terms and conditions of contract should not be worsened before or after the transfer. TUPE legislation is often complex and has come to be applied to downstream production tender processes in television sport.

In 2009, when Niall Sloane, the newly appointed director of sport at ITV, sought competitive tenders to take over production of all ITV Sports' output, a number of companies were asked for proposals. However, the application of TUPE meant the incumbent production team based at ITV appeared to be protected. Consequently, any bidding company had to deliver a cost-efficient production plan at the same time as hiring all of the ITV Sport staff, many of which had lengthy service and subsequent redundancy entitlements. In other words, had an independent production company won a three-year contract to produce ITV Sport output, it could also inherit a substantial financial liability including redundancy settlements. In this case, having obtained a range of competitive quotes, the contract was awarded to the ITV sports production department.

Whilst the logic of TUPE is apparent in the case of the ITV tender (where a whole department may, potentially, have been relocated) this logic is much less obvious in cases where a rights holder decides to tender for *alternative* production services, i.e. when they are seeking a change of direction. In 2012 such a case involved Al Jazeera Sport. The company had content produced by ITV but it now wished to consider alternative producers, so Al Jazeera put its portfolio of production out to tender. With an annual budget of around £7 million this production interested several independent sports production companies. However, legal advisors confirmed that TUPE applied. If the contract were to be awarded to a company other than ITV, then the current production staff (hired by ITV but working on the Al Jazeera contract) would need to be transferred across at the exclusive risk of the new production company and not at the risk of the rights holder, Al Jazeera. Firstly, it is hard to see how production output could be changed substantially if TUPE required the outgoing staff to be placed on the new production. Secondly, the incentive for an independent sports production company, already working on slim margins, is further reduced if TUPE is applied. This is another example where, in theory, the objectives of regulations are fundamentally well intended but, in practice, they fail to make much sense in the circumstances. Since around 2009, TUPE has increasingly been applied to sport production tenders. In another example, when, in 2011, Channel Four acquired the rights to all top-class UK horse racing the production services were put out to tender. However, the winning company had to TUPE-in members of the outgoing production team in order to secure the contract. These cases were corroborated by testimony received from senior executives involved.

Looking at such examples, the evidence suggests there is often a gap between the objectives of downstream supply side regulation and the actual outcomes. In terms of regulation and intervention as applied downstream to the content supply side, then regional production quotas and TUPE can be seen to have had a massive impact on the activities of independent sports production companies and are important but often neglected factors that are shaping the content supply market.

Conclusion

Regulation is the third pre-production factor that influences what sport we can see and where we can see it; regulation can also influence who makes the final programmes. Cultural, social and historic values surrounding sport have, to some extent, been maintained in Europe, but this is under constant threat from the ever-increasing commercial and market-driven activities of leagues and federations, including the Premier League and UEFA. The crucial role of the list of protected list of events was explored, including the adoption of similar protection across the EU. With neither included on this list, interventions against the Premier League and UEFA were reviewed and questions about the usefulness of some outcomes were raised, particularly the impact on the final consumer. In the case of the Premier League, it was EC intervention that brought BSkyB's monopoly hold on broadcasting rights to an end. However, the same intervention caused further inflation in broadcasting fees, benefitting the Premier League.

Although there is no protected list of events in the US, the Major Leagues have maintained a strong presence on the four free-to-air commercial networks and have not migrated to pay-TV. The leagues have also adopted voluntary rules that help maintain the value of their broadcasting rights, including (a) an equal share of television rights to all member clubs, (b) salary caps for club rosters, and (c) a reverse-order-of-finish draft system for players entering the professional leagues. Evens, Iosifidis and Smith (2013) conclude that the increased exposure and higher audience ratings delivered by free-to-air television *can* serve the interests of teams, leagues, broadcasters, advertisers and viewers alike.

Consistent with providing a supply side perspective some ways that regulation *directly* impacts on production practices was discussed including, in the UK, the role of Ofcom in regulating (a) the market, and (b) maintaining production standards. Threats to the values as set out in the Broadcasting Code were discussed. These included an apparent hegemony among sports producers that led to a kind of self-policing of standards, plus challenges from digital media platforms where content is largely unregulated.

This chapter also discussed two regulatory aspects not normally discussed in the literature: the impact on independent production companies of regional production quotas and the impact of TUPE regulations insofar as this can determine who will work on a production when a commission is transferred from one production company to another. The chapter concluded by observing the gaps between the theory of regulation and the practical outcomes found downstream on the production supply side, this was despite the positive intentions that underline regulations.

It was also suggested there was a need for new ways of thinking about regulation in the upstream markets, including looking at (a) the solutions adopted by the US leagues, and (b) increased levels of self-management by leagues and federations to provide a more constructive path forward.

Chapters 3, 4 and 5 examined how largely unseen pre-production processes (including technology, broadcasting rights and regulation) operate upstream. As they interact these processes exert an increasing influence on what television sport looks and sounds like, where it can be seen and who can see it. Unpacking the downstream impact of developments in technology, broadcasting rights and regulation, the focus now turns to a micro-level analysis of the work of broadcasters and media providers, plus the day-to-day work of independent sports production companies.

6
Broadcasters and media providers

Chapters 6 and 7 zoom in to examine how the upstream processes discussed so far impact on (a) broadcasters and media providers (including *who* provides sports media), and (b) independent sports television production, from company-level activities to a micro-level view from the shop floor and the day-to-day work of sports producers and directors. These chapters add a further supply side perspective.

As demand continues to outstrip supply, increased competition to acquire sports broadcasting rights has delivered good economic news for the elite leagues and federations (Fort, 2006:53). The challenges facing broadcasters are now considered including: (a) the increasingly complex relationship between rights ownership and the commercial performance of broadcasters and media providers, (b) the emergence of federation-based host broadcast operations providing 'approved' coverage for major events, (c) how increased demand for sports content has delivered almost no critical comment, and (d) a widening division between coverage and presentation, how rights-holding broadcasters localise and rebrand the coverage provided by federations. The chapter draws on field notes supported by interviews with a select group of key executives, senior producers, directors, heads of production and production managers working for broadcasters and independent sports production companies between 2011 and early 2015.

6.1 Commercial performance and market polarisation

Whilst increased competition to acquire sport broadcasting rights benefits leagues and federations, broadcasters and media providers face a number of challenges, with economics providing an ever-increasing barrier to entry. As sports broadcasting is an oligopolistic market structure it is dominated by large networks (Doyle, 2002); one supplier's actions can have a significant impact on its competitors (Brander and Spencer, 1983). Two elements are of critical importance to all broadcasters: audiences and content. Cottle (2003) provides a useful summary of how the market structure encourages certain types of behaviour:

> This involves an inherent tendency towards media concentration through buying up (or out-pricing and ruining) competitors, processes of vertical integration (extending control over the entire production and distribution processes), and horizontal integration (combining related or complementary businesses) as a way of reducing costs, increasing market share and corporate control. A number of other consequences flow from this same logic of economics. (Cottle, 2003:9)

For Boyle and Haynes (2004) the consequences of opening British broadcasting to market forces included the introduction of full commercial competition in 1992. BSkyB established itself as the dominant player in the UK sports television market as the company amassed a portfolio of the most appealing live sports rights and grew its subscription base. It was only the intervention of EC competition authorities that ended BSkyB's monopoly hold on live Premier League rights. As the dominant force, BSkyB also had a major say in determining new distribution methods; it strictly controls access to its platform, including its EPG and the critical audience data collected.

With the UK's terrestrial broadcasters unable to compete economically with BSkyB no substantial threat was posed by the arrival of Setanta, or when Setanta failed in 2009 and ESPN acquired Setanta's former rights. However, in 2012 the arrival of BT in the UK sports rights market, followed by its two-channel launch in summer 2013, has seen the competition to acquire key sports rights intensify further, creating consequences for both corporations.

BT was motivated to enter the market due to concern the company could lose critical core fixed-line telecoms business, particularly broadband, to BSkyB. Hewlett (2013) speculates BT had £700 million annual revenue at risk. In this case attractive sports content was used to bolster BT's existing services – BT Broadband customers were offered the new BT Sport package free of charge. Garside (2015) confirms BT hoped its sports channel would stop customers defecting to Sky and help grow revenues and profits. BT's consumer division has grown revenue and profits for five consecutive quarters; for seven quarters BT has added more broadband customers than any other provider in the UK.

BT's initial investment of £400 million per year on elite football and rugby union rights was followed in November 2013 by another £300 million per year deal agreed for the purchase of European football rights (UEFA Champions League and Europa Cup from 2015). At £897 million for three years, BT's winning bid is more than double the amount paid jointly by BSkyB and ITV for the previous three year period. Enders Analysis (2013) calculate that, whilst BT can absorb this cost due to the large size of the company, the direct revenue returns through subscription charges and advertising on BT Sport are expected to fall far below the annual rights payment. Whilst BT's initial cost-versus-income equation can be questioned, Garside (2014), reviewing figures for the final quarter of 2013, reports that BT's push into football and fibre broadband has helped deliver a forecast-beating 2% rise in revenues across the BT Group, with BT Sport attracting half a million extra customers (to 2.5 million in total). This suggests the ways the most expensive sports broadcasting rights are being valued is becoming more complex as is increasingly linked to the overall corporate performance of the largest media providers, particularly those with ambitions to provide 'quad-play', a combination of television, broadband, fixed line telephone and mobile services. Owning attractive sports rights is another way of safeguarding their other businesses.

In 2015 BT successfully bid for a further three years of Premier League rights (for seasons 2016–17 to 2018–19, costing £960 million for 42 games per season, a rise of 17% over the previous rights secured). BT Consumer's chief executive, John Petter, defended company strategy:

> There were a lot of sceptics and there were a lot of people who thought we'd somewhat lost the plot in 2012. But the numbers speak for themselves. The consumer business is doing better now than it ever has done. Not only are the profits growing consistently, but even before the investment in sport the profits are up. (Gibson, 2015b)

Managing director of television and sport for BT, Delia Bushell, adds: 'Sport and television are emotional products that really connect in to subscribers. And, if you're a broadband provider, combining the two into a great-value bundle has a real anchor effect', (Midgley, 2015). Midgley (2015) also confirms that in BT's results for 2014–15, full-year revenue for BT Consumer – including retail telephony, broadband and television – was up 7% with the Ebitda [earnings before interest, taxes, depreciation and amortisation] profit measure up 24%. Broadband and TV revenues were up over 16% over the full year. But the transition from telephony to a full pay-TV provider that is launching a third ultra-high definition channel (BT Sport Ultra HD) has not been entirely smooth. Brignall (2013), reviewing Ofcom data, notes that the level of complaints from BT TV customers in August 2013 about the quality of service provided more than doubled and were running at 11 and 28 times the rate of complaints against Virgin Media and BSkyB respectively – half of the complaints were about the newly launched BT Sport channels. Williams (2013) reports the complaints centred on difficulties in receiving the channels. Prior to the launch BT's TV service was already the industry's worst performing in terms of complaints to Ofcom, attracting 6.5 times the average (Williams, 2013).

Recent sports broadcasting rights auctions, including the UEFA Champions League and Europa League matches, plus Premier League rights, highlight the increasing connection between sports rights ownership and corporate performance. With all UEFA Champions League and Europa League matches migrating to BT Sport in 2015 and FA Cup matches to be split between BT and the BBC from 2014–15, BSkyB reported an 18% fall in pre-tax profits (BSkyB 2013; Sweney, 2014b). The company's adjusted operating profits (the figures most closely watched by analysts) fell by 8% year-on-year. BSkyB's share price also fell 2.6%. Ahead of the 2015 Premier League rights auction BSkyB's chief executive Jeremy Darroch is quoted as saying:

> Of course the Premier League is an important set of rights, we get that, we will go in with a clear view of what we seek to achieve. Whenever [the auction] arrives we will be ready and in good shape for the process. With any set of rights there is a price beyond which we don't think it provides value. That was the case with the [UEFA] Champions League. It accounted for just 3% of viewing and there were better ways [to invest]. (Sweney, 2014b)

To some extent BSkyB achieved its goal of retaining five of the seven Premier League rights packages available in the 2015 auction. But it came at a very high cost, £4.176 billion and almost double what the company paid for the previous rights. By comparison, BT Sport agreed to pay £960 million for two packages, enough to attract and retain broadband customers. As a result, around £350 million was reportedly wiped off BSkyB's value, as investors feared the satellite broadcaster had overpaid for the rights. Farrell (2015) notes that shares in BSkyB fell by more than 2% while BT shares rose by 16.2p, or 3.6%. An analyst at Westhouse Securities, Roddy Davidson, concluded that BT had secured the better deal:

It does look like BT has enhanced its competitive position by bouncing its arch-rival into an aggressive bid, while incurring a less dramatic 30% uplift in its own cost base in return for a broadly comparable rights portfolio, retaining a base of Premiership coverage to sit alongside its Champions League rights and, maintaining flexibility to invest in other genres. (Farrell, 2015.)

The acquisition of expensive rights packages soon had further consequences for both media providers. Since entering the market in 2012 BT Sport has maintained that 'for too many years, too many people in this country have been asked to pay too much to view televised sport . . . ' (BT Consumer's chief executive, John Petter, quoted in Garside, 2015). However, in changing its approach of 'making more sport available to more people' (Gibson, 2015b) and offering BT Sport free to subscribers of BT Broadband, BT TV and Sport managing director, Delia Bushell, accepted the offer 'was not as simple' as it was before (Midgley, 2015). Whilst Petter claims the new rights fees agreed are 'a manageable increase on what we've paid previously' and such increases remain 'within the scope of it's [BT] case' (Gibson, 2015b), BT now charge £5 per month to access top-flight European football. To receive all other BT Sports channels for free, from mid-2015 a BT subscriber will have to pay at least £36 per month for a package that includes a set-top box, pay TV, discounted phone calls, line rental and broadband, (Garside, 2015).

Just six weeks after it agreed to pay a record fee for Premier League rights, BSkyB increased its monthly subscriptions, rising to £47 per month for a sports television package. The gamble to retain these rights has also led the company to redress its entire sports strategy. Sky Sports managing director, Barney Francis, presented his view of the way forward, 'Fit for the Future', to staff in April 2015. Plans will see Sky Sports concentrate on their live rights while reducing the support programming and by making savings by not automatically replacing staff that leave the network, (Sale, 2015). BSkyB claim this was a strategy talk, not cost cutting, and is designed to prepare for the varied demands of a multi-platform future where the perceived role of traditional programme making may be diminished.

Despite claims from BSkyB that the company is unwilling to overpay for rights, the coverage of top-flight football has been critical to the growth of BSkyB. Gratton and Solberg (2007:143) suggest that BSkyB risks losing 50% of its subscribers without Premier League coverage. Throughout the 1990s, having spent over 50% of the value of its sports programming expenditure on football (Szymanski, 2006:155), losing any further elite rights may present a major challenge and is likely to lead to diversification in an effort to retain subscriptions. However, with new customers for broadband and Now TV (BSkyB's no contract 'pass' pay service), by mid-2015 BSkyB's UK operation was reporting its best subscriber growth in 11 years, to the end of March 2015 (Sweney, 2015a).

With the remarkable amounts of money involved in acquiring sports broadcasting rights there is increasing amounts of risk and a very real danger of encountering *winners' curse*, of paying too much and the underlying business model failing (Fort, 2006:64). Despite such risks the market is still driving forward, Rankin (2013) notes that the sports rights market grew 14% in 2013, and Deloitte, anticipating the market in rights to hit £16 billion in 2014, sees no end in the rush to acquire premium content with revenue growth driven by new broadcast deals for Premier League football, Germany's Bundesliga and MLB Baseball in the US. The Premier League rights deal for 2016–19 makes it the second most lucrative league just behind the NFL, which generates $4.5 billion each season (Peck, 2015). Increases in sports right payments are forecast to outpace global pay-TV revenues, suggesting that the stakes (and risk) continue to rise. Gibson (2015a) notes that media analysts and City experts have stopped asking when the Premier League bubble is going to burst and now speculate on whether it will continue to defy economic wisdom by continuing to inflate, including changing shape depending who is in the market to purchase broadcasting rights. In market conditions like these, if BSkyB and BT reach the limits of what they are willing to pay, there would be an opportunity for even larger corporations such as Google, Apple or Microsoft to acquire the most appealing sports broadcasting rights and change the content distribution model again (Evens, Iosifidis and Smith, 2013). Matching sport content to technology, particularly in distribution, is a story that appears to be just beginning.

The large portfolio of international rights acquired globally by Al Jazeera (often trading as beIn Sports) is also worth noting. As an international live sports director, interviewed in 2013, points out: 'Al Jazeera, Google and Microsoft could not only buy sports rights, they also have their own technological gateway via their own devices'. As the largest multinational players operate across borders then broadcasting rights could be purchased for key territories, or for all distribution, both UK and international, or even for the purposes of warehousing them. Indicating how quickly the scenario can change, in June 2015 the US broadcasting network Discovery, owner of Eurosport, signed a deal costing £920 million for exclusive pan-European rights to the Olympics

Games from 2022. This deal ends previous arrangements made with a consortium of public service broadcasters across Europe. However, without a change in legislation Discovery will be required to broadcast all Games free to air. As reported by Gibson (2015d) Discovery and Eurosport will help develop a new Olympic channel under the IOC's supervision.

Polarisation in sports content provision

Despite the efforts of media regulators and competition authorities from the UK and the EU, the evidence suggests that only the biggest and best-funded pay-TV broadcasters and Telcos or the biggest transnational corporations are able to acquire live sports rights.

As the battle between BSkyB and BT Sport continues in the UK, the market is effectively split, leaving the contest for major events (where access is ensured via the list of protected events), highlights packages and what might loosely be determined as second tier sports providing realistic targets for the BBC, ITV, Channel Four and Channel Five. However, for the UK's free-to-air terrestrial broadcasters the ability to deliver large audiences and offer a shared viewing experience retains considerable value.

As the BBC competes against well-funded rivals, Barbara Slater, the BBC's director of sport, accepts there is a 'new reality' in the market for live sports rights (Gibson, 2012). Despite the successful presentation of the London Olympics, 2012 was a challenging year for the BBC. It lost its horse racing rights to Channel Four, and, after 10 years coverage, MotoGP rights were lost to BT Sport. It also re-positioned its Formula 1 coverage as a junior partner to Sky Sports. In terms of organisation, when the sports department relocated from London to Salford it shed 43% of its staff. And, as part of the BBC's overall Delivering Quality First initiative, the sports rights budget was cut by 20% (Gibson, 2012).

Slater recognises the disadvantage the BBC carries by having a finite income that, in real terms, is reducing over time. The corporation is also challenged, in so far as it cannot monetise expensive broadcasting rights via subscription charges or by attaching sponsorship or advertising to content in the ways its competitors can (Gratton and Solberg, 2007). In view of the BBC Charter renewal (due in 2017) then the BBC may need to target which rights it can realistically secure, for example coverage of the Wimbledon Lawn Tennis Championships was prioritised over retaining full Formula 1 coverage. In its defence, Gibson (2014b) argues that London 2012 was hugely important in defining the BBC's role as a home for communal viewing in the digital age. The ability to reach large audiences is the BBC's defining characteristic, particularly the presentation of global events.

Recently, ITV has also seen its portfolio of sports broadcasting rights reduced, losing FA Cup coverage and, from 2015, the UEFA Champions League and Europa League. World Cup Finals, for football in 2014 and rugby union in 2015 are the remaining highlights. In 2013 Channel Four acquired broadcasting rights to major horse racing events in the UK. Produced by IMG Sports Media across 90 racing days, 73 are reported to have suffered a drop in viewers over the previous year (Cook, 2014). However, Channel Four received a favourable response to its coverage of the 2012 Paralympics; this represented a considerable commitment to an event that, previously, had not received a great deal of primetime coverage. Viewed in conjunction with the BBC's Olympic coverage, plus world cup finals in football and rugby illustrates the benefits of greater prominence for major event coverage on terrestrial television. Previously absent from the list of broadcasters with major events, Channel Five struck a three year deal with the Football League to air a weekly highlights package in primetime on Saturday evenings, (Sweney, 2015b). The migration of Football League highlights is another loss for the BBC.

Whilst there will be intermittent skirmishes that may yield a sports rights win, or a coverage and/or highlights share with Sky Sports or BT Sport, there is little evidence to suggest the continued migration of live sports coverage towards pay-TV in the UK will slow down. As a senior executive from the BBC but now at a major independent sports producer summarises:

> In the early 1990s the BBC had everything. There were tears in the corridors when rights were lost. Now the [BBC] sports department is much smaller, the BBC has lost a load of rights. A lot of their main stuff is now made by independent producers. Sky has changed the overall view of what is acceptable, Channel Four continues in much the same way and ITV even has its own sports channel in ITV Four. The biggest difference is that there are a lot more people drinking at the fountain, whereas it just used to be one person. (Senior executive, independent sports production, 2013)

Asked to look ahead, a senior manager who has worked at both the BBC and Sky Sports adds:

> I think the World Cup Finals and Olympics will continue on traditional free-to-air television for a long time... Will the World Cup

Finals or Olympics be on Sky Sports soon? No. In 20 years, possibly, but not even in the medium term let alone the short term as the major events are all protected. But this will change. (Senior manager, ex-BBC and BSkyB, 2013)

The entry of Discovery and Eurosport into the market with the acquisition of pan-European Olympic rights is more imminent than anticipated. However, the BBC's director of sport, Barbara Slater, defends the role of free-to-air broadcasters in this quote:

We have got a very peculiar intensity of competition between Sky and BT, leading to extraordinary hikes in price for certain properties. But there is a place for free-to-air. I think you take your sport off free-to-air television at your peril... It's about your new audiences and your future audiences. To create heroes, they need to be seen. (Gibson, 2014b)

Slater's predecessor at the BBC, Roger Mosey, concurs: 'What we showcased in 2012 is that sport can bring the UK together like nothing else, and public service, free-to-air television is essential in doing that', (Mosey, 2015). Attributing the loss of rights held by PSBs to 'soar away inflation caused by pay TV'. Mosey continues:

Imagine [coverage of] London 2012 behind a paywall, with the triumphs of Bradley Wiggins and Jessica Ennis only seen by those who paid a subscription; or contemplate the future of the Champions League now wholly owned by BT or the lessons of cricket only live on Sky. However good a job the pay broadcasters do, public service and maximum access for all are still things that matter hugely in the world of sport. (Mosey, 2015.)

The cornerstone of the BBC's PSB remit – delivering important sporting events to a national audience (Boyle and Haynes, 2000:69) – is echoed by Slater and Mosey. Slater claims that while BBC Sport accounts for 2% of sport output in the UK it attracts 40% of the viewership (Gibson, 2014b). What the 40% of viewership watch is not specified but is likely to include major events that benefit from the shop window effect the BBC still offers. However, as the BBC faces further scrutiny of the value it provides for £3.5 billion leading into the charter renewal this is a critical period. Gibson (2012) notes that cuts to BBC sports presentation draws concern from powerful sports organisations, including the IOC and The Royal and Ancient (organisers of the Open Golf Championship), both of which have agreed future rights deals with Discovery and BSkyB respectively, so what other sports choose to remain committed to the BBC despite its access to larger audiences is an increasingly serious issue.

But this is not the only challenge. The influence of a small group of specialist advisers and, particularly, the advance of federation-based coverage of major events are significant developments.

A small world: special advisers

A consequence of the current intensification in competition for the most appealing sport rights is the apparent reliance on a small group of, mostly male, advisers. Selling its broadcasting rights, the Premier League has received advice from specialist firms including DLA Piper and Reel Enterprises (part of the Wasserman Group since 2011). The current BT Sport chief Marc Watson previously worked at Reel as a *seller* of sports rights. Watson is now a *buyer* of rights for BT Sport (Sweney, 2012). The list of executives attributed with operational knowledge of the sports broadcasting rights business includes a number of former BSkyB executives: Sam Chisholm (who negotiated the original Premier League deal for the newly merged BSkyB), Dave Hill (who became CEO of the Fox Sports Media Group after leaving Sky Sports) through to recent BSkyB CEO Tony Ball. Having left BSkyB, Ball, hired as a non-executive director, then advised BT on its sports rights acquisitions including the Premier League. Additionally, there are legally trained rights negotiators including Simon Johnson, formerly of ITV Sport who subsequently joined the Premier League. Whilst the increased activity in specialist consultants is broadly in line with corporate activity, the movement from one side of the table to the other – primarily from television sport to senior positions at the leagues and federations – provides evidence of how boundaries are becoming more fluid.

For example, two people I have worked with include former controller of BBC Sport (and former Channel Four sports commissioning editor) Mike Miller, who, after leaving the BBC, spent 10 years (until 2012) as chief executive of the International Rugby Board (IRB). Miller is attributed with negotiating rugby union's inclusion in the 2016 Olympics and is now chief executive of the World Olympians Association. Similarly, the Football Association (FA) turned to a former controller of BBC and ITV Sport, Brian Barwick, as its chief executive between 2005 and 2008. In January 2013, Barwick became chairman of the Rugby Football League, again suggesting that sports federations value senior managers with direct broadcasting experience. As broadcasting is often a primary source of revenue this makes sense.

However, an entirely new phase in sports television production is associated with television executives moving to federations. Bernard Ross had been an executive producer with IMG Sports Media working on the early stages of the Premier League's international output, plus major event international coverage for FIFA and UEFA. In 2006 Ross joined UEFA as head of TV production, to plan and implement the host broadcast of UEFA EURO 2008. This was the first time UEFA had taken the television production of the tournament in house to produce the international feed. This was a significant step.

Also of note is John Rowlinson, previously a senior executive at BBC Sport. In 2002 Rowlinson moved from the BBC to the All England Lawn Tennis Club (AELTC) at Wimbledon before becoming its director of television. In 2009 Rowlinson was hired by the London Organising Committee (LOCOG) of the 2012 Olympics as head of broadcast for the International Broadcast Centre (IBC). The IBC was the home of Olympic Broadcast Services (OBS) during the Games and was the base for around 15,000 media workers linked to rights-holding broadcasters (Sweney, 2009b).

In the small world of television sport an even smaller group of power players has emerged where a few male, mostly former television executives have come to wield a considerable amount of influence. One of the most significant steps is for federations to take charge of the television coverage for their own events, rather than depending on local national broadcasters to provide this service.

6.2 Federation-run host broadcast operations

Since around 2005 FIFA, the IOC and UEFA have set up their own host broadcast operations for major sports events, replacing the role previously held by the host nation's national broadcaster. The line between what is best for the sponsors and advertisers wooed by the federation's promises of sympathetic coverage and the final television output *also* provided by the federation is neither straight nor straightforward. This significant development is now considered.

At all major global sports events, the International Broadcast Centre (IBC) is a bespoke technical and broadcast hub used for broadcast operations and rights holding broadcasters (RHBs). Coverage of each individual event is routed to the IBC's central media servers where content can be accessed by rights-holding broadcasters before being uplinked to their respective territories for broadcast. The International Broadcast Centre model can be viewed as an extension of the Premier

League Productions workflows and UEFA Champions League Production Manual conditions discussed in chapters 3 and 4.

Funding for the planning, construction, engineering and equipping of the IBC is provided by the local organising committee (LOCOG) and/or Olympic Delivery Authority (ODA) but can also be privately funded, either way the costs are not carried by the IOC or FIFA. Gibson (2009) places the cost of the 2012 London Olympics International Broadcast Centre at £355 million.

OBS, IOC and OTAB

Olympic Broadcasting Services (OBS) is based in Madrid. Created by the IOC in 2001, the company specialises in covering multi-sport events according to its website: 'to serve as the host broadcaster organisation for all Olympic Games, Olympic Winter Games and Youth Olympic Games', (OBS, 2013). The explanation continues:

> The Host Broadcaster is responsible for delivering the pictures and sounds of the Olympic Games to billions of viewers around the world. It produces and transmits unbiased live radio and television coverage of every sport from every venue. This feed is called the International Signal or the World Feed.

> In this role, OBS is responsible for developing a consistent approach across Olympic operations while at the same time optimising resources to continually improve the efficiency of the Host Broadcast operation.

> OBS does so to ensure that all IOC contractual obligations are fulfilled and the Games' Rights Holding Broadcasters (RHBs) are satisfied with the overall television production of the Olympic Games. (OBS, 2013)

Local broadcasters are no longer responsible for providing coverage, although they may, as sub-contractors, still contribute to the overall OBS operation. It can be argued that the main beneficiaries are not the rights-holding broadcasters, but the IOC's highly developed programme of preferred global sponsors – TOP. Consequently, the extent to which OBS coverage can be considered unbiased is open to question. In terms of providing coverage that is sympathetic to sponsors and advertisers, then, the role of Olympic Broadcasting Services introduces another level of control on behalf of the IOC by removing an *intermediary*, the local broadcaster. A senior producer who worked on several Olympics looking after international output for the IOC explains the role of digital technology in allowing Olympic Broadcasting Services to take control of operations:

> Between 2000–2004 we had access to all IOC content, we made the programmes, including highlights, and sent them out to the RHBs [rights holding broadcasters]...By 2008 OBS [Olympic Broadcasting Services] via their central server at the Beijing IBC had total control. Everybody now worked under the OBS umbrella. Everything is done according to the Manuals you are given; it's all pre-conceived so you have very little leeway in what you can possibly produce. I would place the watershed for this change at around 2005. (Senior sports producer, independent sports production, 2013)

To better understand this critical shift we need a benchmark. Prior to 2005 the IOC contracted IMG Sports Media to provide international production services for rights holding broadcasters. Between 2000–04 IOC library managers at IMG would receive feeds of all event coverage routed from the venues, Sydney and then Athens. A senior sports producer involved in production picks up the story:

> The feeds would come in; they would be recorded onto digital tape where they would be logged so that producers could find what they wanted from the library. From 2008, and Beijing, the operation had gone entirely digital. There was a big server in Beijing, everything was fed into that and all rights holders could come and pick up what they wanted. Tape storage was no longer relevant. (Senior sports producer, independent sports production, 2013)

It was a similar story with FIFA and Host Broadcast Services (HBS) as an executive producer with significant major event experience recalls:

> The first time I encountered central media servers at a major event was the 2006 World Cup Finals in Germany. Rights-holding broadcasters had a meeting each day where Host Broadcast Services (HBS) would say what was available in the central pot. The technology has been around for a while – it was around in Japan and South Korea in 2002 – Host Broadcast Services will be in charge again in Brazil 2014. (Executive producer, independent sports production, 2013)

By the middle of the decade federations had taken charge of host broadcast operations and, using central servers and digital workflows, produced an international feed to be used by all rights-holding broadcasters.

For the IOC there were two important outcomes: 1) the IOC, via Olympic Broadcasting Services, now had much more control of its own material, including how the coverage looked, who could access it and a detailed log of what material was used, and; 2) the IOC no longer needed to contract a company like IMG Sports Media to carry out its international production operations, although IMG was retained to run the Olympic Television Archive Bureau (OTAB). OTAB manages the commercial processes of licensing Olympic footage and all IOC symbols. As the OTAB website says:

> Ultimately we are involved with your project from the conception of your ideas to the final cutting stage, so we can service all your requirements from sourcing of Olympic content, the licensing and rights clearance stages to the final approvals of the production. (OTAB, 2013.)

The OTAB explanation is indicative of increasing supervision and approval processes for the use of *all* IOC material.

Returning to Olympic event coverage, Olympic Broadcasting Services subcontracts production of each Olympic event to individual specialist producers, or to national broadcasters that may have expertise in specific event coverage. So, for the London Olympics the BBC becomes one contractor (albeit a large contractor) among others that were hired by Olympic Broadcasting Services to cover the entire range of events and to produce a sympathetic feed with consistent production values. The removal of national host broadcasters from *coverage* of Olympic events leaves them free to focus on the *presentation,* or localisation, of the Games for their own national audiences.

To illustrate the extent of control exerted by Olympic Broadcasting Services an example from 2008 came to my attention. A senior producer, a fluent Mandarin speaker, and an executive producer who were in Beijing working on the Games corroborate this account. In 2008 the best canoe slalom director had twenty years' experience of covering the sport and was based at Slovenian television. The director, Stane Skodlar, and his team were brought in by Olympic Broadcasting Services to cover the white water canoe slalom event at the Beijing Games. However, Skodlar was presented with an OBS manual explaining exactly how to direct the slalom coverage. With no room given to interpret these instructions the director's expertise was redundant, although his name was still attached to coverage that, in his words, 'could have been directed by anyone'. Conversely, and again through experience as a participant-observer, in 2013 I was aware of a senior producer attributed with coverage of the dressage event at London 2012. When IMG hired this director to help with a proposed dressage event in Qatar it turned out that his knowledge of outside broadcasts and directing the event was limited – apparently he had followed the instructions provided by Olympic Broadcasting Services in their manual for dressage coverage.

Whilst the television departments at the IOC, FIFA and UEFA are now far more instrumental in defining exactly how productions should look and sound – as expressed in their detailed production manuals – at least some senior television executives believe that federations cannot do everything themselves:

> Federations do now get control over their events, but they still need to hire people to do the production work for them. The federations will determine how it is seen, where it is seen and how much they charge. But they still need cameramen and directors [to cover events]. (Senior executive, independent production, 2013)

In other words, the federations require producers hired on short-term contracts (preferably assured by companies like IMG or a recognised national broadcaster). But, with the need to comply with the specifications set out in the manuals and so deliver approved coverage, the function is increasingly one of painting by numbers. It should also be noted that federations increasingly police the quality of final coverage provided to ensure it complies with the requirements set out in the production manuals. A senior manager with extensive experience working for broadcasters at major events concludes:

> Some Olympic events, like the marathon, will always look different because the setting changes every four years. But for many other events, yes, they are all becoming more prescriptive. (Senior manager, independent sports production, 2013.)

An experienced live sports director adds:

> The Olympics gives a very clear instruction about what is and is not allowed … It's all linked to commercial obligations as sport becomes more commercialised. Federations and organisations need to protect

those relationships and that's one way of doing it. (Live international sports director, 2012)

Increasing prescription and conformity is the price of the IOC seeking totally dependable television coverage.

Another aspect of the dependability of international television coverage is more prosaic, but also a factor. This involves providing clear cue points throughout the broadcast timeline, so that rights-holding broadcasters, working in different time zones around the world, can opt in and out of the international feed when they want to. This is a very similar procedure to the UEFA Champions League Production Manual's multilateral running orders discussed in Chapter 4. Directing live sport to a defined and pre-determined timetable whilst adapting to unpredictable outcomes within these parameters leaves little or no leeway for interpretation. No surprises are required.

According to all the expert contributors interviewed, the outcome is an Olympic television product that is subject to increasing control by Olympic Broadcasting Services on behalf of the IOC. This television product receives an injection of local colour and tone every four years but, essentially, the aim is to achieve consistency, avoid controversy and any surprise material that would offend or otherwise compromise sponsors and advertisers spending significant sums to be associated with the Olympic movement. With no advertising allowed inside Olympic venues – unlike perimeter advertising in football – the IOC, according to a senior producer with experience of three Olympics and related in 2013 'are desperate to avoid ambush marketing in and around the stadia'.

Given the production prescriptions and preferred methods now set out by Olympic Broadcasting Services, it appears to make less and less difference who actually directs event coverage, whether it is individuals, independent production companies or national broadcasters with specific expertise. Since the mid-2000s the use of new digital technology has provided the IOC and Olympic Broadcasting Services with a quantum leap forward in their ability to control much more of their own output.

The rise of the global sports event was discussed in Chapter 2, but looking at the Olympic movement since Sydney 2000, Magdalinski *et al* (2005), argue that the Games now represent the incorporation of sport into multinational advertising and marketing strategies. They state:

> This partnership between sponsors and the movement has solidified the rapid process of commodifying the Olympics as a 'product' and

has established a clear link between the future success of the Olympic movement and leveraged its ability to attract capital funding from external supporters. (Magdalinski *et al*, 2005:46)

Recalling Gruneau and Cantelon (1988:347), the Olympics has been transformed into an increasingly market-oriented project where there is 'a more fully developed expression of incorporation of sporting practice into the ever-expanding marketplace of international capitalism'. In practice, this can be reduced to (a) taking control of television output to provide dependable and sympathetic output suitable for consumption worldwide, and (b) the ability to exclude any and all material that might in any way compromise the IOC or TOP members. The IOC is now the gatekeeper and its own regulator.

HBS, FIFA and UEFA

UEFA took significant steps to extend its control of coverage of the Champions League and Europa League via the production manuals it issues as a key part of broadcasting rights agreements (see Chapter 4). In comparison to multi-sport events like the Olympics, top football tournaments feature a single sport with a limited number of games – Brazil 2014 featured 64 matches – so, in many respects, they present slightly less challenging logistical circumstances. Television output from international football tournaments, including the FIFA World Cup Finals and the UEFA EURO Championships is now supervised by each federation's television department working with Host Broadcast Services (HBS) in ways similar to Olympic Broadcasting Services on behalf of the IOC.

Host Broadcast Services (HBS) was founded in 2000 and is fully owned by Infront Sports and Media, a sports rights and marketing company based in Zug, Switzerland. The Infront company profile claims it is 'helping to transform the industry' (Infront, 2013:1) by 'targeting sport at the core of an ever growing and widening matrix of the entertainment industry' (Infront, 2013:3). The inclusion of sport as another element of the entertainment industry is not in question (Whitson, 1998; Boyle and Haynes, 2000). Host Broadcast Services (HBS) was established to produce the television and radio output for the 2002 and 2006 FIFA World Cups. On the HBS website the company profile page states:

HBS is responsible for producing the multilateral coverage and providing unilateral production, transmission, commentary facilities and associated services for world broadcasters at the FIFA World Cup™. To achieve this, HBS designs, builds, installs and manages an

International Broadcast Centre (IBC) and the multilateral and unilateral broadcast facilities at every venue in the host country. (HBS, 2013)

Host Broadcast Services influence has increased since the 2006 FIFA World Cup Finals in Germany. The objective is to take control of every aspect of production, 'from pitch to the active viewer' (Infront, 2013:15). Host Broadcast Services seeks to control everything to do with the international feed and its distribution globally via satellite. To paraphrase: work begins with an audit at the venue to establish local resources and delivery needs. Host Broadcast Services is responsible for planning, building, managing and dismantling the International Broadcast Centre as well as providing the multilateral and unilateral on-site broadcast facilities at all venues (HBS, 2013). In addition to the international feed the unilateral requirements of rights-holding broadcasters including unilateral production, transmission, commentary and on-site production services (such as editing and archive provision) are provided by Host Broadcast Services. HBS also provides what it intriguingly calls 'knowledge management' as well as 'legacy archiving'. This is simply information and media archiving activities undertaken when the organising federation does not already provide these services.

In comparison to the Olympics, a World Cup Finals tournament generates around 120 hours of football, so the volume of media should be easier to manage (although by the time various match feeds, isolated camera angles and EVS feeds are added this volume increases dramatically). An innovation pioneered by Host Broadcast Services is embedding an individual producer with each World Cup Finals team. The HBS producer works exclusively with the assigned team to access news stories and provide profiles, features, interviews and updates that will be made available to all rights-holding broadcasters via the central media server for use in their own presentation as required.

Hidden from immediate view is how Host Broadcast Services and Infront now operate *together* to control many critical aspects of event staging and television presentation. Reviewing HBS and Infront websites, plus Infront (2013) their activities embrace:

- Event positioning, brand development and promotion.
- Individual company sponsorship strategies.
- Event management, venue dressing and signage, including LED venue advertising solutions.
- Hospitality, catering, accreditation and ticketing services.

- Media rights sales.
- Coordinating broadcast coverage and digital asset management, including longer-term archive management and clip sales.
- Creating digital communications platforms for media, brands and products.

Recalling Patrick Nally's influential *Intersoccer* template (Nally, 1979), since the mid-2000s FIFA and UEFA, working closely with Host Broadcast Services, have taken decisive control of all aspects of major international football tournament coverage. As has been the case in other examples, from the Olympics to Premier League Productions, it is a combination of factors that have enabled this move, including: (a) powerful media servers, (b) the ability to move large amounts of media between locations, (c) the capacity for numerous rights-holding broadcasters to access the same source material simultaneously, (d) to produce and distribute different outputs, and (e) the ability of federations to provide approved coverage of their own events for international consumption (via localised presentation provided by rights holding broadcasters). An important part of approved coverage is guaranteed protection and enhancements for key sponsors and advertisers.

Considering the rapid development of the host broadcast operations by Olympic Broadcasting Services and Host Broadcast Services, in addition to new content distribution models – like the Premier League's full channel service available in more than 200 territories, plus excursions into bespoke broadcast channels by the NBA and NFL (with both organisations retaining established production arms in *NBA Entertainment* and *NFL Films*) – there can be little doubt that the downstream television operations provided by the leagues and federations has entered an important new phase. The precise relationship between these new federation-run television operations and competition authorities and media regulators remains unclear.

Reviewing developments in conjunction with a perceived lack of accountability on behalf of the IOC and FIFA, and fed by allegations summarised by Jenkins (2014), raises serious questions about purpose:

> These organisations' staff travel the world like heads of state. They require more lavish facilities and kowtowing. They must stay free at hotels, be greeted by presidents and prime ministers, have armies and navies on hand to guard their ceremonies, and have domestic markets rigged for their sponsors' products. Roads must be closed for their limos and traffic lights phased to green. The politics of host

nations are of no concern to them. No one calls these bodies to account, because they claim a higher licence from the great god of sport. (Jenkins, 2014)

Falcous (2005) identified a triangular alignment of corporate, media and sport interests and how this accelerated phase has resulted in sport being linked with more instrumentally rational approaches to capital accumulation. But, where do these developments leave broadcasters?

6.3 More scope, less criticism; even more media, and coverage versus presentation

Considering the challenges facing broadcasters engaged in fierce competition to acquire sports broadcasting rights at the same time that federations have taken control of producing their own international feeds, three trends are worth reviewing: (a) whilst the volume and scope of output has increased dramatically, criticism (of leagues and federations) remains minimal, (b) as yet more content is provided, broadcasters engage with viewers via the red button, online and second screen applications, and (c) the widening split between coverage and presentation in television sport.

More scope, less criticism

Even a brief review of channel schedules suggests that *all* broadcasters are engaged in eking out as much value as they can from their sports broadcasting rights. Sky Sports, for example, has its own strategy department dedicated to maximising value under an overall 'vision to be the world's best sports business'. Looking across sports television output in 2015 it is apparent that a much wider scope of output has emerged, this now includes:

- Live sports coverage.
- 'As-live' sports coverage (coverage routed through EVS with several minutes delay built in, i.e., NFL coverage on Sky Sports).
- New made-for-television sports (*Fight Night, UFC, Premier League Darts*).
- Magazine presentation (live, as live and highlights usually presented via a studio, for example from the 2013–14 season *Match of The Day* offers a third edition).
- Stand-alone highlights (usually sport-specific, like Ashes Test cricket).
- Weekly review and preview programmes.

- Discussion formats (some formats featuring a panel of journalists, others with players, ex-players and coaches).
- Sport-celebrity vehicles (Sky One's *In a League of Their Own* and, previously, *Jumpers for Goalposts* plus the BBC's *They Think It's All Over*).
- Traditional sports quizzes (BBC's *A Question of Sport*).
- Sport-celebrity feature programmes (access-based lifestyle films. Trace Sports offered a whole channel of lifestyle-oriented content).
- Sports documentaries (from Sky's *A Year in Yellow*, to one-off films on ITV 4 and a specialist documentary strand on BT Sport).
- Fanzine formats (*Soccer AM* and *Fantasy Football*).
- Archive-based formats (*Premier League Years*, *Football Gold*, *Football's Greatest*, *Sports Greatest*, *Premier League 100 Club*).
- Personality interviews (often ad hoc and offered around a product launch).
- Chat shows (host plus guests, previously BBC's *On the Line*).

Sky Sports News has a dedicated channel with its own signature event, the closing stages of the football transfer window. Within football coverage general discussion is not limited to the Premier League and its fixtures, but is focussed more specifically on mini-leagues *within* the league – for example, the race for the title, the battle for European places, bragging rights in local derbies and the fight for survival (the avoidance of relegation) at the bottom of the league. This has been noticed in research:

> But even in an unequal league, like the Premiership, our results imply that the modern creation of 'leagues within leagues' permits many games to generate extra interest because they 'matter' for some issue or another. (Forrest, Simmons and Buraimo, 2006:99)

With 154 matches broadcast per season between 2013–16 (116 on Sky Sports and 38 on BT Sport) creating reasons to watch is not surprising. However, generating more scope can involve adopting overtly entertainment-based production values, the BBC's *Sports Personality of the Year* provides an example. In the early 1990s, when the BBC still retained the majority of sports rights, the popular annual review programme was titled *Sports Review of the Year*. Subsequently the programme was rebranded and on 15 December 2013 it celebrated its sixtieth anniversary. The new format is a glittering sports-celebrity-awards show, complete with an entertainment style floor and lighting rig. The sports action clips are sourced from a variety of broadcasters.

The crossover between sport and entertainment has also generated a range of celebrity-sports-entertainment formats. These are often prominently positioned in schedules and include:

- *The Jump* (Channel Four), a celebrity contest based around several winter sports first aired in January 2014 ahead of the Sochi 2014 Winter Olympics (BBC).
- *Splash* (ITV) a celebrity diving challenge featuring 2012 Olympic bronze medalist Tom Daley also broadcast in January 2014.
- *Dancing on Ice* (ITV) featuring Winter Olympic gold medal winners Torvill and Dean, broadcast in early 2014.
- *Tumble* (BBC) a celebrity gymnastics format launched in summer 2014, featuring 2012 Olympic silver medalist (and BBC *Strictly Come Dancing* champion) Lewis Smith and Nadia Comaneci, the first gymnast to score a perfect 10 in competition.
- *Olympic Superstars* (BBC) a specially staged television tournament post-2012 Olympics aired as a Christmas special (Channel Five re-launched the IMG owned *Superstars* format in 2008).
- *The Match* (Sky) a celebrity versus retired professional footballers challenge match ran for three series with additional support programming.
- *The All Star Cup* (Sky One), a celebrity version of golf's Ryder Cup.
- *Famous and Fearless* (Channel Four), eight celebrities in a multi-extreme sport challenge broadcast in early 2011.

In purely economic terms there is some appeal to creating formats that do not incur the considerable rights fees attached to elite professional sports events. If successful, these new formats can be reformatted for international sales generating further income. Usually made by entertainment producers, these formats are not considered as replacements for regular weekly sports coverage but act more like special offers used to attract viewers to the channels, somewhat like special events including Olympics (Fikentscher, 2006:85).

Whilst the scope of sports television output has increased substantially, critical comment is harder to find. The few programmes that might hold FIFA or the IOC to account are distanced from sport output and broadcast under current affairs strands like BBC *Panorama*, including a campaign against FIFA corruption by the journalist Andrew Jennings – see Jennings (2006) and Simson and Jennings (1992). More typical of the current climate is an example from January 2013, when ESPN issued a statement implying that one of its commentators, Jon

Champion, had wrongly labelled a Liverpool player, Louis Suarez, as a cheat for using his hand in a live FA Cup match. Champion said: 'That, I'm afraid is the work of a cheat' (Gibson, 2013). ESPN, which was in the third of a four-year deal to show FA Cup matches, distanced itself by adding:

> We take our responsibility to deliver the highest standards of coverage to our viewers. ESPN's editorial policy is for commentators to be unbiased and honest, to call things as they see them. Inevitably this can involve treading a fine line on occasion, especially in the heat of the moment. (Gibson, 2013)

Evidently, such lines are even finer when important sports broadcasting rights are due to be renewed. Limited discussion of some issues – like foreign ownership of football teams, player wages, Financial Fair Play Regulations or even constantly changing kick-off times – can be found on radio particularly via listener phone-ins. However, comments still may not draw much of a challenge: on 22 December 2013, the Premier League's chief executive, Richard Scudamore contributed to Gary Richardson's BBC Five radio show. Asked to outline Premier League activities in 2014 Scudamore said the first priority would be to 'protect the Premier League's intellectual property rights worldwide'. Scudamore did receive some scrutiny in May 2014 when emails he wrote containing sexist comments were released. However, despite dominating the agenda elsewhere, Sale (2014) reports the story was practically ignored by Sky and News International newspapers. The FBI's intervention in the investigation of FIFA in spring 2015 was primarily covered by mainstream news, providing banner headlines for several days as arrests and further revelations were made. However, in general terms, as television's protection of the culture of sport serves to maintain the hegemonic position it enjoys with sport, so Boyle and Haynes (2000:107) see an obvious reason to avoid criticism: television knows 'that it must not kill the goose that lays the golden eggs'. For Perelman (2012) the situation is even worse:

> We are not just witnessing an increased mediatisation of sport, but mediatisation deployed – *decreed* – by sport itself, in whose influence the media is steeped through and through. (Perelman, 2012:89.)

From a Marxist stance, Perelman sees sport as having expanded across the planet leading to its successful and nearly complete globalisation –

as 'an irresistible power it has no equal' (Perelman, 2012:109). With all critical positions excluded from mainstream discussion: 'sport as an institution today is the vanguard of non-criticism', (2012:110).

Even more media

Another contemporary trend sees broadcasters emphasising alternate means of viewing their sports content. In some ways this is part of a pattern where ever more volume and scope of content is offered. Various forms of content linked to innovative means of viewing can also be used by broadcasters as a point of differentiation in their marketing manifestos. This content also represents further commodification of sport as a media product (Boyle and Haynes, 2004).

Enhanced or interactive viewing essentially falls into three areas:

- *Additional* coverage that supplements the primary channel output, usually broadcast behind the red-button accessible via a TV remote control. Content ranges from adding a cockpit camera in Formula 1 to alternative match choices for football such as Champions League on Sky Sports.
- *Associated* content streamed on the Internet, usually via a linked website, and ranging from clips to lengthy streams of events, for example choice of coverage from multiple courts during Wimbledon or from more specialised Olympic events, like Judo.
- *Second screen* or social media; a range of dialogues taking place parallel to the main coverage. Twitter, for example, is used by broadcasters to give the appearance of being connected to their audiences.

Particularly since London 2012, the BBC has offered what director of sport Barbara Slater describes as the 'deeper experience' for viewers (Gibson, 2014b). Slater argues that viewers want the communal, shared moments of seeing big event coverage live on television, but they also want an option to customise their experience and 'go deeper' via online access. For the Sochi 2014 Games two interactive streams were available behind the red button and six more streams on the BBC video player available on all viewing devices. The BBC sees this added value as a major point of difference it provides to viewers.

For BSkyB enhancements such as on-demand, Sky Go, and its EPG interface have been drivers in creating customer loyalty and form a significant part of the company's promotional activities – 'expect more' to quote a 2014–15 campaign phrase. As discussed, BT Sport, via its fibre broadband services, is making a case for converged media. Doyle

(2002:20) argued that, ultimately, there will be no difference between broadcasting and telecommunications. However, the extent to which these services have taken off is open to question.

Illustrating the apparently slow take up, the idea of immersive viewing was introduced first by Sky Sports, as an experienced live director explains:

> In terms of immersive and social viewing, Sky Interactive did this 10 years ago, by offering a choice of different camera angles via the [television] remote control. Viewers could access statistics and Hawkeye too, so that's all been around as an enhancement for a while. The new thing is 'talking about sport', are viewers interested in what other viewers are saying? More people are checking this out before expressing an opinion. (Live sports director, Sky Sports, 2012)

The option to use match choice via the red button is well established and a consequence of greater capacity in the digital spectrum. As part of sports presentation, the inclusion of Twitter and Facebook, for example, on top of SMS and email, has risen substantially since 2010. But just how important or relevant this may be is open to debate; a respected executive producer with broadcaster and independent sports experience offers this view:

> 90% of all viewing is still via television. Digital and mobile [consumption] is still only one in 10 people – I think this will continue for a long time. World Cup Finals and Olympics will be on traditional free-to-air television. Twitter, connected TV and so on, it's really important in pitches, but come the interview it never gets mentioned, broadcasters want to know what we will see on the main screen. Broadcasters pay lip service, but I think they know in their heart of hearts what drives this business. (Executive producer, broadcaster and independent production, 2013)

To what extent the current preoccupation among broadcasters with alternative means of delivering content and generating viewer discussion is a passing fashion or is part of a genuine shift towards convergence and more customised viewing habits remains to be seen as there is simply not enough evidence to draw any meaningful conclusions at this time. In addition to the difficulties in raising revenue from these new platforms an experienced senior producer expresses a widely held view among producers interviewed and one that reflects the dramatic increase of scope in sports content more generally:

> I'm not convinced you can slice up events much more. The Olympics is different as it has so much [action that] you might want to see it all... Formula 1 cockpit cam, no one is really bothered, or different angles of football coverage you can choose from your own seat, but covering football *differently*, that might be interesting. (Senior sports producer, independent sports production, 2013)

As the organising federations define match coverage at major football tournaments, any significant changes appear unlikely. But, how many more ways sports content can be recycled and re-broadcast is a relevant question; it is also one that federations have been considering. According to an executive producer at a large independent sports production company speaking in 2013: 'it is certainly not clear that federations have, so far, fully grasped the dynamics of this new landscape'. That leagues and federations are unclear about how they want to engage with newer aspects of digital media tends to fuel confusion. I have first-hand experience of how leagues and federations can be very clear about many of their production activities (via production manuals), but away from primary coverage and website support they are much less sure about how to proceed – e.g. online, on social media. Following a tender for production services in late 2012 the IOC decided to experiment with their own dedicated *YouTube* channels during 2013. The IOC decision came from its marketing department suggesting such activities are part of promotional strategy rather than fully integrated with their broadcasting plans.

Returning to broadcasters, with output largely defined (a) by the rights a broadcaster holds, (b) coverage of major events provided by the federation, and (c) due to an increased volume of sports coverage originating in other countries and re-broadcast in the UK – for example, Spain's La Liga, Germany's Bundesliga and Italy's Serie A – broadcasters face a further challenge in differentiating their product as they move from providing original coverage to offering 'wrap around' presentation of events.

Coverage versus presentation

The *presentation* of television sport, as distinguished from its *coverage*, is a development worth noting. There has been a substantial increase in sports covered by one party – a league, federation or a local broadcaster –

that is broadcast (essentially re-broadcast with embellishments) by another. The Olympics offers an example. As noted, Olympic Broadcasting Services, rather than the national broadcaster from the host country now provides coverage of the Olympics. For the BBC this means it has been able to focus more effort and resources on the presentation of the event.

In addition to commentating on the coverage provided, the additional shoulder programming – including *all* presenting and reporting around the event – is an increasingly important aspect of broadcast output as it seeks to both localise and brand the generic international coverage provided by the federations. The precise division between coverage and presentation can be difficult to see as broadcasters like the BBC typically have access (in their rights agreements) to additional unilateral feeds within the arena (in other words, to cameras under the BBC's direct control that may be used to track specific UK interest, like a featured athlete) and they will certainly have cameras for their own presentation positions and for post-race interviews.

Although the change in emphasis from coverage to presentation may suggest limitations, or even a degree of passivity, wide variances in presentation style are easily found. For example, the BBC adopted a fairly catholic view of the Olympics, reporting widely on a whole range of events and competitors; it seeks to provide a reasonable overall picture. This contrasts sharply to NBC's presentation in the US. In my experience of viewing Olympic coverage in the UK and the US, the focus in the US is almost exclusively on US athletes. US presentation style often amplifies human drama and emotion (a story might report on a competitor who has recently lost a parent and dedicates their performance to this memory). These feature stories are highly produced, and, with coverage mostly time delayed to fit US network prime-time schedules, an altogether more personal narrative is presented, mainly to the exclusion of stories that have little or no US interest. In general, it is a narrower angle of view. For London 2012 NBC was widely criticised in the US for its approach as many viewers already knew the results via Internet access.

The BBC underlined its commitment to presentation by securing prominent studio positions at London 2012 and, before that, in Cape Town for the 2010 World Cup Finals. In a main point of difference with the BBC's London 2012 semi-open studio vantage point, and use of exterior links in the Olympic Park, Channel Four chose a fully *enclosed* studio that did not provide the same immediate connection to the venue seen on the BBC. For Sochi 2014, it was noticeable that the BBC opted for an even more agile and informal presentation style with presenters linking from a variety of completely open locations – it was a more immersive style compared to a formal and closed studio presentation. A brief look at football (particularly UEFA Champions League) and rugby union coverage (on Sky Sports and BT Sport) reveals a trend for using pitch-side positions for at least part of the main programme presentation.

More generally, the primary presenters – the faces of an event like the Olympics – are carefully chosen, with teams of reporters and experts added to the onscreen line-ups. Although not responsible for coverage *per se*, the BBC had production teams of 295 at the 2010 World Cup Finals (Gibson, 2010) and a team of 765 for London 2012 (Gibson, 2012b). Presenting London 2012 to its UK audience, the BBC spent approximately £66 million (Sherwin, 2014).

The critical importance of determining presentation style is underlined by the intervention of Channel Four's chief creative officer when the final composition of the on-screen presentation team for coverage of the 2012 Paralympics was changed *after* the press launch and extensive screen testing (as relayed, in 2013, in an interview with a senior producer who was at the launch and involved in subsequent discussion).

Away from major events, more and more sports are bought in by broadcasters and presented via a studio, usually featuring a host and relevant guests – again, localising non-UK originated coverage for viewers. With four dedicated Sky Sports channels devouring 672 hours of content a week – joined by a fifth channel in August 2014, a further dedicated channel for Formula 1 and 'pop up' channels devoted to special events, like Ashes cricket – the necessity of bringing in additional content is apparent. Interviewing sports producers in 2012 and 2013 provided a snapshot of how many popular sports are now *presented* rather than *covered*. For example, European Tour Golf is covered by European Tour Productions, a joint-venture company owned by the Tour and IMG Sports Media. The same team produces Ryder Cup coverage when the event is held in the UK. For tennis, the ATP World Tour (the governing body of men's professional tennis circuit) has its own broadcast operation that provides an international feed to over 110 rights-holding broadcasters, including BSkyB. Popular European football is covered by local broadcasters, including La Liga on Sky Sports, with the Bundesliga and Serie A carried by BT Sport. And NFL coverage comes from BSkyB's sister company Fox Sports and the other rights-holding US broadcasters that provide game coverage.

Presentation style was also a major selling point in the BT Sport launch, with promotional trailers featuring BT's large studio (previously the international broadcasting compound for the 2012 London

Olympics and used by Channel Four for the Paralympics) – virtually all of the launch trailers featured action specially shot in this distinctive space. Glendenning (2013) quotes BT Sport's director Simon Green: 'Without getting personal, the presentation of football hasn't come on a huge amount in the last 15 years. We [BT Sport] think we'll bring something different'. At the end of two seasons of Premier League football any differences appear to be rather nuanced. In addition to the central hub design of the studio with its prominent monitor banks, the only innovation was the use of a small live box sometimes inserted in the corner of replays so nothing is missed during the time the replay is on screen. In the conservative world of television sports production even relatively minor changes are often lauded as innovative.

Considering these brief examples, whilst more effort and resources are put into presenting sport, it is evident the main point of difference between broadcasters is the portfolio of sports rights that each holds. However, as major event coverage is increasingly provided by federations, with leagues issuing ever more detailed prescriptions for coverage and the need to fill a high volume of broadcast hours on multiple channels with additional sports content, then the individual presentation style each broadcaster chooses to adopt is important, not least because it remains one of the very few areas for which they still retain substantial control and, as such, has become a key part of their channel brand.

Conclusion

This chapter reviewed a range of challenges faced by broadcasters following upstream transformations in technology, broadcasting rights and regulation. Challenges included: (a) the close relationship between sports broadcasting rights ownership and the commercial performance of large media firms, (b) the emergence of federation-based host broadcast operations providing 'approved' coverage for major events, (c) how increased demand for sports content has delivered very little critical comment, and (d) a widening division between coverage and presentation, how broadcasters focus on localising and re-branding the international coverage they receive from federations via individual presentation and branding styles. The chapter maps the continuing flow of power upstream, away from broadcasters and towards the leagues and federations.

Examples from BT Sport and BSkyB were used to examine how the commercial performance of media providers is linked to ownership of popular sports broadcasting rights. In an oligopolistic market structure, changes in sports broadcasting rights ownership can directly impact on the economic performance of competing companies; the growing significance of corporate performance also suggests the way in which sports broadcasting rights are valued is becoming increasingly complex and risky. With the migration of many sports rights to BSkyB and BT Sport, a split in the market providing sports content was reviewed, including the possibility on encountering *winners curse* and bidding too much in a market where rising prices for broadcasting rights shows little inclination of slowing down.

Further challenges for broadcasters arise as a result of (a) the influence of a small group of mostly male special advisers many of whom have moved from executive positions in television sport to work directly for the leagues and federations and (b) the emergence of federation run host broadcast operations; Olympic Broadcasting Services and Host Broadcast Services in particular.

Enjoying commonalities with Premier League Production workflows (Chapter 3) and the Production Manuals and shared international feed philosophy adopted by UEFA (Chapter 4), the IOC, FIFA and UEFA seek to take control of *every aspect of production* to provide a dependable and sympathetic international feed to all rights holding broadcasters. In doing so, the line between what is best for advertisers, sponsors and broadcasters becomes more blurred. Research by Gruneau and Cantelon (1988) and Magdalinski *et al* (2005) notes how the Olympics have become 'a more fully developed expression of incorporation of sporting practice into the ever-expanding marketplace of international capitalism', (Gruneau and Cantelon, 1988:347). This book argues that federation-based production is a very important new phase in television sports production.

Considering the significantly increased demand for sports content, including more volume and scope, and the introduction of formats that embrace more entertainment-oriented production values, there remains very little in the way of criticism in sports television output reflecting a reluctance to 'bite the hand that feeds', (Boyle and Haynes, 2000:107).

The provision of *more* media is a central theme as broadcasters try to engage viewers via the red button, online, mobile platforms and second screen activities (such as peer group dialogues). Whether this is a marketing exercise by each channel (providing added value), or indicative of a shift towards more customised viewing is unclear as there is insufficient evidence to reach a conclusion. It was noted that federation activity in this area is comparatively underdeveloped.

As broadcasters respond to increased league and federation-based production activity that delivers approved coverage to all rights holding broadcasters, plus an increase in coverage originated by other broadcasters and bought in to fill schedules, then the importance of *presentation* in sports television has increased significantly. Whilst the BBC faces intense commercial competition to acquire rights for protected events like the Olympics and World Cup Finals, the corporation has, with the rise of federation-based host broadcast operations, been released from providing comprehensive *coverage* of events. This has allowed the BBC to concentrate its efforts and resources on the *presentation* of major events, in other words the shoulder programming that wraps around international coverage and that serves to localise it. Presentation is also a means to differentiate broadcast output and to build a brand identity. Presentation is one of the remaining areas where broadcasters still retain substantial control. Although the BBC retains a plausible position as the broadcaster that can deliver a shared viewing experience for large numbers of British viewers, this has not prevented the corporation from losing a significant amount of rights.

Continuing to offer a supply side perspective that charts the impact of pre-production process downstream, Chapter 7 examines contemporary trends in independent sports production and the day-to-day work of sports producers and directors.

7

Independent sports television production

Subject to considerable upheaval as pre-production processes have trickled down to the supply side, the television sports production workplace can be a confusing environment. On face value it might be reasonable to assume the transformations reviewed so far could have been the foundation for a creative heyday for sports producers and directors. In some important respects a very different scenario is playing out, one that is shaped by inhibitions and restrictions. This chapter examines trends in independent production, from investment in production companies through to the rise of the production manager.

Academic research describing the contemporary day-to-day work of sports production companies, producers and directors is scarce. Among a limited and dated output – Barnett (1990), Whannel (1992), Boyle and Haynes (2000, 2004) and Haynes (2005) – observations by Tunstall (1993) remain useful. Developing an idea put forward by Burns (1977) Tunstall argues that producers operate in 'closed and private worlds', (Tunstall, 1993:2). This is accentuated by working within prescribed genres that serve 'to shut sports producers off from the rest of the world of television' (1993:67), for sport, the distinguishing features include high volume of output, unscripted content and technical complexity amongst others. This chapter argues that important new sub-genres *within* sport further delineate production skills, for example, the emphasis placed on live coverage, and this creates more pressure to specialise. Tunstall also questioned whether the prominence placed on technology and logistics in television sports diminishes its journalistic value (Tunstall, 1993:72). This updated account sees prescriptive control as one of the major issues faced by independent sports producers and directors.

7.1 The UK independent sports production sector

The first UK independent sports production companies emerged in the 1970s and 1980s; the launch of Channel Four in 1982 was significant, as was the 1990 Broadcasting Act, as it introduced a general independent production quota of 25% across all non-news commissioned programming (HMSO, 1990; Mediatique, 2005). In sports production, the growth in sponsored and bartered distribution content (where programmes are typically provided to a broadcaster for free in return for advertising space) and collaborations directly with federations, for example the joint venture between The European Tour (of golf) and TWI (now IMG Sport Media) to form European Tour Productions in 1991 also added impetus. However, the UK independent sports production sector has never been large. Over the past two decades some companies have ceased trading and the remaining firms shifted orientation from focussing on creative output to realising their value as a business, with a corresponding tendency to offer more specialised output. On the nature of markets, Doyle (2002) writes:

> The structure of a market depends not only on the number of rival sellers that exist but on a variety of other factors, including differences in their product, the number of buyers that are present, and barriers to the entry of new competitors. (Doyle, 2002:8)

The UK independent sports production sector remains small and the entry of new firms, like Endemol Sport in 2009, is relatively restricted (Khalsa, 2012).

Background

Cheerleader Productions was one of the first independent sports production companies in the UK. I worked at Cheerleader from the late 1980s, the company was funded by an annual fee it received from Channel Four (around £400,000 per year, as relayed by the managing director), for which a team of six producers and assistant producers were on call, effectively acting as the Channel Four sports department. Managing director, Derek Brandon, also confirmed Cheerleader policy was to adopt an overtly US-styled approach to production values, arguing that televised sport in the UK was under-produced compared to US sports productions. Methods and technologies were freely imported as Cheerleader packaged US sport for UK broadcast including the NFL. I was producer of Sumo, added in 1988 for Channel Four, and recall that the process of producing programmes generally took precedence over business affairs, although questions surrounding rights and other issues, including specified access at events, were beginning to impact on production work.

An ex-ITV and BBC executive, Mike Murphy, set up Television Sport and Leisure (TSL); the company bought and sold sports rights in what was a fledgling market. During an interview in 2011, a senior production manager that worked for TSL confirmed that Murphy began to offer production consultancy, again a new area for independent producers, including selling the overseas broadcasting rights to the 1991 Rugby World Cup.

Founded over 40 years ago Trans World International (TWI, now IMG Sports Media) was established as a part of IMG to add television production services for clients the McCormack organisation already represented, including golf and tennis federations. Interviews with sports producers working for TWI in the early 1990s confirm the company began to specialise in outside broadcast coverage from challenging locations. Equipment was designed for packing and transportation between venues, including island hopping for West Indies cricket and league football from China. Whilst TWI pioneered flyaway production techniques, from May 1987 it also produced the long-running magazine, *TransWorld Sport*. Speaking in 2013, one producer who graduated from *TransWorld Sport* to Chinese football recalls there was 'still a tendency for broadcasters and federations to view different cultures through sport'. This was certainly the case with early Channel Four productions from *Sumo* to *Kabaddi*. The producer also added a note about prominence: '[before multi-channel sport] what it does mean is people remember better and were more attached to sport when there was less of it [on television]' (Series producer, independent sports production, 2013).

Using sport as a lens to view culture was a relatively short-lived approach as the downstream market in sport content provision began to change in the early 1990s. The same producer suggests that, pre-dating the expansion of BSkyB in the UK, the Pan Asian satellite channel, Star, was the first dedicated sports channel to require significantly more sports content to fill its schedules. In the US ESPN and TBS also required more content. In changing market conditions TWI was well-placed to react. From the outset, and due in part to the background of several of its senior executives, TWI was often viewed as a sort of annexe to BBC Sport – in early 2014, three out of four of the company's most experienced executives had prominent BBC backgrounds. Some senior IMG producers speaking to me in interviews between 2011 and 2013 confided they saw the company as the 'Marks and Spencer of sports television', because it provides competitively priced programmes, including large volumes of content, rather than stand out creativity and innovation. That IMG represents federations and rights holders and has sales offices in numerous countries is also significant. A former ITV head of production, interviewed in 2013, confirmed a widely held industry view that IMG provides a benchmark for costs: 'You always get a production quote [price] from IMG as this will give you a guide to the lower end of expected costs on any project'.

The UK's independent sports production companies were small but each, in some way, was pioneering. Sunset + Vine was formed in 1983 to produce sponsored/advertiser-funded programmes and offer bartered syndication deals, like *Gillette World Sport* that ran for 25 years between 1984 and 2009. Interviews with programme producers confirm that distributed magazine programmes like *Gillette World Sport*, *TransWorld Sport* and *FIFA Futbol Mundial* saw their access to elite content dramatically restricted with the extension of sports broadcasting rights and copyright control – 'We just can't do top level sport anymore; the rights are prohibitive and exclusive', (Series producer, independent sports production, 2013).

Cheerleader Productions split in 1989, with Derek Brandon and several colleagues joining event entrepreneur and former athlete Alan Pascoe to form Grand Slam Productions, where advertiser-funded content was targeted. In response, the original Cheerleader Productions brought in an executive producer from the BBC, Charles Balchin, as the company continued to produce NFL and Sumo coverage into the early 1990s before the Daily Mail General Trust (DMGT) purchased it.

In the early 1990s Chrysalis fully entered the independent sports production sector. Chrysalis Sport Managing director Neil Duncanson confirmed he took advantage of an opportunistic moment when making a documentary on Paul Gascoigne – the England player who had famously cried during an Italia 1990 match and had been transferred from Tottenham to *Serie a* club Lazio. To show any Italian football highlights in the Gascoigne film Chrysalis had to acquire the broadcasting rights to *Serie a* from RAI, the Italian broadcaster and rights holder. The acquired rights were offered to Michael Grade, then at Channel Four, who purchased them in 1992 just as BSkyB had acquired exclusive rights to live Premier League football. Significantly the *Gazzetta* weekly highlights programme was complemented by live coverage on Sunday afternoons, as *Football Italia* became the only live league football that could be seen on terrestrial television in the UK. By looking for gaps where they could operate in the content production market, independent sports production companies had already taken the first step towards specialisation.

Issues

A major problem for independent sport production companies is that they very rarely hold any broadcasting rights. Also, they do not have direct access to audiences. Instead, and unlike general programme provision, independent sports production companies offer services for costs plus a percentage fee to broadcasters or rights holders. Typically, broadcasters will pay all production costs but, because they only hold primary rights, there is no benefit from selling this coverage to other broadcasters (as secondary rights are normally retained by the issuing league or federation, see Chapter 4 for an explanation of primary and secondary rights and Doyle, 2002:80–90). In these circumstances, sports production companies find themselves constantly competing to win production tenders – Request For Production (RFP) and Invitation To Tender (ITT) – issued by broadcasters, federations or third-party rights holders; they are in competition with other independent sports production companies and, sometimes, with broadcast sports departments including ITV Sport.

Independent production companies seldom carry major capital investment in property, hardware and technology, with IMG Sports Media providing an exception with its studios, post-production and satellite distribution divisions located near Heathrow Airport in London. The worth of an independent sports production company is usually based on its production order book, the ability of key staff to attract new business and its potential for growth, with these factors weighed against staff salaries, rents and other operating costs. As a participant/observer I recall managers/owners complaining – at various times when favourable interest rates on deposits were available – they could achieve better returns by putting their money in the bank than investing in independent sports production – a good return was considered to be 3–5%.

During the past decade there has been a trend where private equity firms have taken ownership and shareholding control of independent sports production companies. For example, Tinopolis/Vitruvian Partners control Sunset + Vine and All3Media/Permira own North One. In December 2013, Forstmann Little sold IMG Worldwide to William Morris Endeavour and Silver Lake for $2.3 billion, having purchased IMG in 2004 for $750 million (Sweney, 2013). In May 2014 Discovery and Liberty Global paid £500 million to take over All3Media, including North One (Sweney, 2014). For investors including an agency (William Morris) and a broadcaster (Discovery) sport production is often one arm in a bigger group of independent producers including genres that hold valuable secondary rights to content – as Doyle (2002:82) notes, it is the retention of secondary rights by producers that has attracted venture capital to independent production. However this does not apply to independent sports production companies, as a broadcaster or media provider will hold primary rights whilst the leagues and federations retained secondary rights. At Chrysalis, I heard the owner, Chris Wright, state on several occasions it was 'useful to have a high profile independent sports producer on the books' because boardroom executives often enjoyed talking about Formula 1 and *Serie a* football.

Using my experience working at Cheerleader, Chrysalis Sport, Endemol Sport and IMG Sports Media, and corroborated by field notes and interviews held with senior executives from these companies, the contemporary situation can be paraphrased like this: Today, private equity firms typically work on a three- to five-year business plan that aims to maximise the value of the company before selling it on for a substantial profit. This generates pressure to raise revenues and reduce costs, particularly staff costs. However, given the cyclical nature of sports broadcasting rights and the fluidity in the downstream programme commissions market, plus ever-reducing profit margins (particularly pressure on costs plus fee service contracts that specify a production fee based on a percentage of the overall costs – since the late 1990s these fees have been gradually eroded, typically from 15%, to 10% and now, for larger contracts, where the fee can be limited to 5%), longer term growth planning becomes more challenging. In 2012 the BT Sport RFP identified a number of exclusions, including studios and outside broadcasts, against which no production fee could be charged. When the requirements of regional production quotas, including establishing regional offices, and Transfer of Undertakings (TUPE) regulations – when staff can receive protection if projects migrate from one company to another – are all added, then substantial financial returns become harder to deliver.

Another problem is one of scale. The smaller size of independent sports production companies, at least compared to broadcasters and other media providers, means typical economies of scale and economies of scope enjoyed by broadcasters and large transnational media providers are mostly missing and this can introduce a degree of instability, particularly with expansions and contractions in the workforce. Of all the UK independent sports production companies perhaps only IMG Sports Media, as it seeks to vertically integrate production, studios, post-production, satellite services and distribution, plus access to federations via its agency, rights and archive management services, comes close to this template. Speaking to the managing director in 2013, even a company of this size remains vulnerable to losing its biggest contracts as productions are retendered. Efforts to retain existing contracts and to win new contracts are continuous and costly. Projecting profits, controlling cash flows and managing the company head count have become essential day-to-day activities. At IMG Sports Media in 2013 there was a monthly editorial board meeting for senior production staff. Having attended several of these meetings myself the primary focus was not on editorial matters but on company performance and potential results, a monthly financial health check that is indicative of the current climate. The transformation of independent sports production to a vehicle for private equity investment is part of neoliberalisation, what Harvey (2005:33) describes as 'the financialisation of everything'.

Without direct access to audiences, it can be argued that independent sports production companies exist around the fringes of the broadcasting economy, allowing broadcasters, leagues/federations and sponsors to hire specialist services for costs plus a fee over a longer or shorter term as required. As federations provide host broadcast operations for their own events, then there is a trend for independent companies to act like agencies offering specific production skills and named producers and directors to the market.

7.2   Live television sports production, creativity or prescription?

Since 1992 live broadcasting has come to dominate the UK's television sports landscape, including the work of independent sports production companies. Live sports production has attained a similar level of prominence to that enjoyed in the US, as one experienced producer explains:

> US television sport invented replays, graphics and the use of statistics among other things. These techniques have been exported all round the world now. Sky Sports has adopted very US-styled techniques. Some sports have taken ideas from the US and used them to their own advantage but, overall, we've come a very long way from the way we used to do things in the UK. (Senior producer, independent sports production, 2012)

How far we've come from the way we used to do things in the UK is an interesting point as it signifies the scale of transformation in television sport. One senior manager at an independent sports production company, considered a pivotal point to be ITV's 1978 'snatch of the day' (when ITV acquired football league rights from the BBC):

> You could feel it [the arrival of more money] in the air. Now, the income per head generated by football is comparable to the NFL when market size is taken into account. (Senior manager, independent sports production, 2013)

This underlines the view, held in the late 1980s and early 1990s by football club owners and the newly formed Sky Sports, that television sport in the UK, particularly football, was under-produced. The rapid introduction of up-scaled live production methods and how this took precedence over more traditional presentation, like highlights and magazine formats, represents a very significant change in UK television sports production culture; this gear-change favoured producers and directors that were most comfortable with the technical, logistical and editorial requirements of live broadcasting. Producers and directors that worked on live flagship sports output became the most highly rewarded in sports production. This replicates the status enjoyed by live producers in the US. With large segments of unscripted presentation and studio-based discussion, plus the uncertainty of outcome surrounding matches and events, the demands on producers and directors working in a live environment were significantly different from those working with highlights, magazine formats and documentaries. Live sports coverage is an environment where the ability to think quickly in reaction to events and to manage output, virtually always under pressure, is highly prized. Live production was not so much a new sub-genre but had become *the* genre that defined television sports production.

However, the introduction of more technology in live sports production tends to obscure some important underlying issues. Priorities for live sports directors are often split; a leading international live sports director describes the need for situational awareness and the tension between (a) telling the story of the event, (b) controlling the available technology, and (c) providing a coherent output:

> I need to be aware of what's happening in the match/event and to tell that story. But I also need to be aware of the television environment,

the camera placement and other points of view and how I am putting this together on air. (Live international sports director, 2012)

Live sport production can be an intense working environment. Interviewing a number of live sports directors, it was noted that further tension may arise depending on who the director is working for; is the director required to provide a safe pair of hands when delivering federation-based international coverage, or is something more creative required by a broadcaster for its local audiences? With the dramatic technological changes in coverage that were being rolled out, directing was also becoming more complicated; a live sports director explains:

> Cricket was covered with about eight cameras and four tape machines, now we use twenty-five cameras and eight channels of EVS – the equipment has become much more capable. Since the 1990s we've moved from 48 to 168 inputs into the switcher [mixing desk], one graphics source has become three graphics sources. The size of the kit is small, but the capacity is so much greater. Tape has gone and the advent of servers is simply revolutionary... with an all-digital environment the scale of outside broadcasts has increased hugely. (Live international sports director, 2012)

The introduction of digital technology gave live sports directors significantly more cameras, a variety of graphic tools and considerably more instant replays. These additional inputs had to be managed at the same time as capturing and reflecting the ebb and flow of the story from the field of play. Another interesting point from the interviews concerned creativity and how creative coverage does not appear to be determined by the number of cameras but by the overall way resources can be combined, as a very experienced live sports director testifies:

> It isn't so much the number of cameras used – whether it is eight or thirty-eight – a decent director can use seven cameras and still deliver good coverage. The bigger step changes are replay systems and graphics. EVS allows you to isolate nearly every single camera and choose from 20 different replays. A single penalty incident can generate seven or eight different angles you can discuss later in the pub. Graphics have been transformed from Letraset [a transfer process] on black and white magnetic strips that were keyed in, to what we have now: fully animated team sheets and other match details [statistics]. Don't forget, it wasn't long ago that score clocks didn't exist now

they are taken for granted. (Live sports director, independent sports production, 2013)

Whilst most live sports directors tend to be technically rather than editorially oriented, it is important that technology itself is not the key factor but rather the ways in which this technology is used. Live directors may debate the merits of different technologies and how they have shaped output but they were not the only people to see how this was transforming coverage, leagues and federations saw opportunities to harness new technologies and workflows so they could take production under their direct control. What is interesting is how new digital technology with the dramatic increases in capacity described by directors could certainly be used creatively. However, the same technology also provided the circumstances where federations were able to demand a more prescriptive approach to coverage of television sport.

With the potential offered by a fully digital workflow, this era might have delivered more creativity and innovation but, whilst there have been many enhancements to coverage, issues to do with prescriptive control and standardised output are recurring themes. Nearly every sport can provide some example of improvements in event coverage, from highly mobile flying camera rigs down to miniaturised cameras improving access, plus a wide range of revealing replay and analysis tools. However, there is another crucial non-technical factor that dictates each and every working context, including what can and cannot be done: the *customer* the production company, producer and director is working for. And this influence may be even more significant than the technology used, Haynes (2005:10) goes as far as to say that intellectual property rights have been used to 'actually inhibit innovation and creativity'. The gloss of new technology applied to television sports tends to obscure such issues.

7.3   Commissioning content

As the volume of televised sport content has grown so, too, has the importance of who commission this content and why. The implications of commissioning are now reviewed.

Whilst Tunstall (1993:67) considered that producers were cut off from the rest of the world of television, he noticed a further difference with sports producers:

> ...these producers' world is less private than that of other producers in one important respect. These producers are closer to their

audiences than are the producers in any other genre. (Tunstall, 1993:76)

Tunstall continued to argue that sports producers were unusual in believing that feedback from friends and acquaintances can be helpful. This appears to be based on a strong emotional commitment to sport shared by both producers and viewers (Tunstall, 1993:76). It also raises a relevant question – who is the sports producer's customer?

Historically, as Tunstall found, many producers, as sports fans themselves, have considered their customer was the audience. Doyle (2002:8) reminds us that 'media content has no value unless it is distributed to an audience' and, again (Doyle, 2002:80), that producers are linked to the audience via intermediary stages in a vertical supply chain, therefore it is not the audience *per se* but the broadcaster, federation, or, in the case of advertising-funded programming, a sponsor that is the customer for television programming. This is important because each customer has quite different demands and priorities. Unlike broadcasters, that have some influence via the substantial fees they pay for rights, independent sports production companies are dependent on these commissions for their survival and can easily be caught between the different requirements of rights holders and broadcasters. How this impacts on companies and individuals is now reviewed.

Broadcasters

Since the late 1980s broadcasters have been a critical source of business for independent sports production companies. When a broadcaster wins sports broadcasting rights a further competitive tender may follow. As noted, independent sports production companies are invited to respond to a Request for Production (RFP) or an Invitation to Tender (ITT). When BT Sport launched in 2012, the media provider did not have a substantial production department that could meet its production requirements, therefore it tendered its Premier League football production. As a publisher/broadcaster, Channel Four carries out tenders for all of its major productions. The BBC has regional and independent production quotas it must achieve, whilst Sky Sports occasionally tenders specialised productions, like fishing. Winning these tenders is a critical activity for independent sports production companies.

From 2009, an increased influence from procurement specialists and internal legal and contractual professionals working for broadcasters was reflected in the tender documents issued, particularly in examples from ITV and BT Sport. Increasingly, tenders are set out in such a way that the responses can be scored by the issuing procurement managers with the answers to key questions, the range of services provided and the value measured and then compared. This process is designed to deliver a more rational means of allocating a production contract. Interviews with senior executives at independent sports production companies between 2011 and 2013 suggest they take a prosaic view to responding in so far as 'every box must be ticked' and 'all questions answered' in each tender response, even if this means submitting a final document that can exceed 300 pages without including budget forecasts. It can be argued that the use of scoring to assess the creative aspects of a response is indicative of how creativity has been subjugated in respect to an overall desire for compliance and financial value. However, when it comes to providing evidence then a trend towards specialisation is easier to identify, both at the level of independent sports productions companies and among producers and directors.

For example, having produced Formula 1 for ITV Chrysalis Sport expanded its motorsport expertise to include production of the World Rally Championships and Isle of Man TT. In late 2013, the company (now North One) used this experience to secure a five-year contract to produce MotoGP motorcycle racing for BT Sport (Considine, 2013). Whilst this may be commercial opportunism, broadcasters do appear to be more comfortable where there is a clear track record of production in a specific sport, in this case motor sport. Looking at other examples, Sunset + Vine have been successful in their presentation production – their work around the shoulder of event coverage – including Channel Four cricket, BBC horse racing, Sky Sports rugby union and BT Sport (football and rugby union). By contrast, with a track record of working directly with leagues and federations, IMG Sports Media executives, interviewed between 2011 and 2013, recognise whilst the company is associated with a more conservative outlook it enjoys a reputation for reliability when delivering content. However, the trend is towards providing expertise in any given televised sport production with overt pressure to do so. In 2012 when IMG Sports Media responded to a tender from Channel Four to produce the channel's horse racing coverage, a senior executive confirmed the priority:

> The first thing you have to do is to go for the expert in horse racing. Similarly, to win the BBC snooker contract you have to present people who are known for these sports. Independents have to pitch with expert [producers] otherwise you won't get in. It's like a hamster

running on a wheel, it never changes. (Senior manager, independent sports production, 2013)

This raises the question of whether *replication* has become more important than *originality*; asked how new ideas could be introduced in such circumstances the answer was:

> The funnel is getting narrower. I once totted up how many different sports I had worked on; it came to 42. I don't think this will happen to anyone in the future. Federations are becoming more prescriptive in their production requirements and producers are becoming more specialised [in their output]. (Senior manager, independent sports production, 2013)

The requirement to provide production experts coincides with a perceived narrowing of the funnel for creativity. But these developments also illustrate the increasing division between coverage and presentation in sports television. A factor driving this trend is how federations have taken control of host broadcast operations. Whilst this provides a further opportunity for independent sports production companies to offer their services for hire, what are the implications?

Federations

A respected international live sports director explained the primary differences when producing live content directly for a federation before onward delivery to broadcasters:

> For a federation I'm creating a generic world feed. The premise is guaranteed uniform and stable coverage of the event for all international clients. For the ATP [Men's professional tennis] this would be [for] 138 countries. The world feed follows a set format, so a safe pair of hands is most important as this allows clients [international rights-holding broadcasters] to jump in and out of our coverage cleanly when they want to. It's proper coverage, but safely done. Working for a broadcaster, or a specific channel, would need more creativity, as you are more responsible for how that channel looks and feels. (Live international sports director, 2012)

There are two dynamics operating; between providing standardised international coverage that multiple broadcasters can cut in and out of and more specific coverage designed for a single broadcaster or channel.

A further tension exists around the preference to work for a federation or a broadcaster. Speaking to a number of independent sports producers there was only one who preferred working for a federation; the general sentiment is that federations including Formula 1, UEFA, FIFA and the IOC are increasingly prescriptive in their production requirements. It is argued that this represents a very significant shift from previous working practices of creating a production (usually for a single broadcaster that offered some leeway in interpreting events) to a contract-driven delivery process involving highly prescribed content designed for multiple international users. This is a new kind of content that is nearly always for federations and it contains different levels of compliance within the prescribed workflows and deliverables. Offering a wide-angle view of the situation, a company director at a leading independent sports production company observes:

> Creation [in future] will be around shoulder programming; pre- and post-kick-off, that's where it will come from. Once you go to the stadia and the referee blows the whistle, or the green light goes in F1, whatever, it [the coverage] will be more prescriptive. There is more and more prescription [from Federations] and less and less input from producers. Yes, that's the case. (Senior executive producer, independent sports production, 2013)

These prescriptions include the ways coverage of events are now set out by leagues and federations via their production manuals, with broadcasters taking responsibility for their domestic presentation of the event, in other words the shoulder programming around the event.

Delivering increasingly prescribed content presents its own challenges but, ultimately, it is a more mechanical process (and one that is more easily described in contractual terms as the services provided) than is the case when interpreting events or providing more creative programming. The clarity provided by such prescriptions may suit some sports producers and directors, but by no means all, particularly those used to having more input. A very experienced senior producer summarises:

> Production for the Olympics is by the book. There are excellent producers and directors sitting around with nothing to do other than follow the Production Manual that is provided [by Olympic Broadcasting Services]...The Olympics want to give a product they can depend on – for example with clear cue points [for opt-outs and opt-ins] and good quality. This is how it is sold to rights-holding broadcasters.

The television departments at UEFA and FIFA are also far more instrumental in how it works. At the last EUROs [2012] it was rubbish [for coverage] to go to a top shot immediately after a goal, even before a replay on camera two. It was straight out of the manual 'cos everyone did it. You need to have two or three regular replays before a top shot makes *any* sense. (Senior producer, independent sports production, 2012)

Similar complaints were levied against the prescriptions required in Formula 1 coverage. Some coverage requirements (the sequencing of cameras and replays in particular) do not make sense to directors who have produced their own coverage in the past. Looking at typical prescriptions provided by other federations, a highly regarded sports director adds further perspective:

The Olympics give you very clear instructions about what is and is not allowed. Overt pressure from sponsorship has always been there. It's in proportion to the size of the event – the magnitude tapers down with the organisation running the event, say from the Olympics to the Asian Games. But even small events now give guidelines on what they want and don't want to see. It's all linked to their commercial obligations as sport becomes more commercialised. Federations and organisations need to protect those relationships and that's one way of doing it. (Live sports director, freelance, 2012)

Such instructions increasingly seek to provide television coverage that is wholly sympathetic to the needs of the federations' own marketing and sales strategies, including their relationships with sponsors and advertisers – in some important ways television sports coverage has become another marketing tool for elite sports federations. In Chapter 2, NBA commissioner David Stern was quoted:

That's the beauty of television. Other brands have to buy their way on through advertising. Our core product is a two-hour commercial [the NBA game] that someone pays us to run. (Jay, 2004:229)

Sport as a brand, as a product, and with games and events running as if a commercial, is part of the growing global marketisation of sport. Following work by Whitson (1998), Falcous (2005) argues this type of development:

... represents a new stage in the commodification of sport, such that it may be gradually detached from meanings based on attachments and loyalties. In the place of, and supplemental to, geographical loyalties come the discourse of personal and consumer choice. (Falcous, 2005:59)

It is argued that sports producers and directors *must now play by the rules, or they don't play at all.* As the rules are frequently set by rights holders and apply to broadcasters, independent production companies and individual producers and directors this is a critical point. It is one of the most fundamental changes in television sports production since 2005.

As the rules of the game continue to change, producers were asked what the main difference in working for a federation or for a broadcaster was. A live sports director provided this summary:

The difference is like living in a democracy and living in North Korea. If you are covering an event for a broadcaster you do so from an outside perspective. But, working for a federation, who owns their own rights, the event must be covered in a positive light regardless of how it may seem. Working for a broadcaster gives you that independence to call a spade a spade. But working for a federation you have to tread very carefully and always portray things in a positive light. (Live international sports director, 2012)

Working for federations, producers and directors must always present events 'in a positive light *regardless of how it might seem*' and, by doing so, they deliver approved international feeds (that are sympathetic to sponsors requirements) subsequently aired by rights-holding broadcasters. But, are broadcasters able to act any more independently? In February 2014, it was alleged that BT Sport dismissed ex-referee Mark Halsey as a pundit following pressure from the Premier League (Sale, 2014b). Looking at developments more generally, any serious notion of broadcaster independence appears to be an idea that is in rapid retreat due to the eye-watering amounts of money paid for exclusive broadcasting rights and the subsequent need to comply with collateral commercial relationships. In any case, it is argued that the differences between working for a federation or for a broadcaster have become less pronounced and that, without any significant changes in prospect, many remaining differences will continue to diminish over time. Given the description (by a senior manager at an independent sports producer speaking in 2013) that 'the funnel continues to narrow' another trend within television sports production is evident, the pressure on individual sports producers and directors to specialise.

7.4   The trend towards specialisation in sports production

In November 1997 I worked for Chrysalis Sport where I wrote an internal management document titled *People, practice and profit*. At that time the company had 42 people working on seven major sports productions involving all UK broadcasters. The document explained typical progression through production roles. As independent production is already a form of specialisation, and as companies also have less scale and scope, it is worth providing a brief update as part of a discussion on how specialisation has accelerated. It is also worth recalling Tunstall as he argued the role of television producer does not constitute a profession – there are no recognised qualifications, nor is entry to the sector controlled (Tunstall, 1993:203). The requirements for the role are subjective and dependent on the working context, a context that has been transformed in recent years.

Up to the late 1980s and early 1990s, progression at traditional broadcasters like the BBC and ITV was described anecdotally as filling dead men's shoes, opportunities for promotion mostly occurred when someone left or retired. Junior staff would join as librarians or as trainee production assistants (later known as assistant producers). Staff would be encouraged in one of two directions, towards an editorial role (producer) or towards directing, with a further distinction made between outside broadcast direction and studio (presentation) direction. At the BBC and ITV the engine room of sports coverage, particularly for major events, was the corps of assistant producers who turned around all incoming VT feeds for use on air. With limited opportunities for promotion, breaking out of the assistant producer ranks was challenging. However, as an ex-BBC executive producer speaking in 2013 confirmed: 'The BBC had everything [in terms of rights] so there were opportunities to work on a wide range of sports, from the Olympics to World Cup Finals'.

The arrival of independent sports production companies, followed by BSB (Champion), Sky and then BSkyB created more fluidity in what had been a very static job market. Changing demand also placed a greater premium on producers and directors with live broadcasting experience.

Entry level at an independent sports production company was as a runner, researcher or even as receptionist. Junior assistant producer was the next step, someone that could carry out action editing: provide basic scripting, location contacts/fixing and short feature storytelling. Senior assistant producers would shoot and edit complete features and be able, under supervision, to construct shorter format programme episodes. A junior producer would do much the same, but with slightly less supervision, whilst a producer would take charge of a complete programme working under a series editor/producer or an executive producer.

A series producer would take charge of multiple programmes in a strand, manage the team and ensure all paperwork and archiving is completed. A series editor differs in so far as they would provide an overview for studio-based productions featuring guests and discussion. Heading the team is the executive producer, someone that selects staff for each project and works on a number of series simultaneously, providing more advanced programme development and detailed project planning, including preparing responses to competitive tenders from broadcasters or federations.

For live sports television, gaining relevant experience can be challenging, even more so for freelance contractors. Some vision mixers have progressed to become directors, but another route would involve an assistant producer running replays, the multiplexer (a machine used to route VT signals to the studio), or switching a number of live isolated cameras into a single feed. Access to opportunities improved if you were assigned to a single sport and could build up a reputation as someone that could be trusted. Beyond that there may be limited occasions to provide second unit direction, or a small OB providing a live inject to a larger programme. A step up would be for lower specification coverage from an 'as live' minor event.

Training in television sport is primarily on-the-job, with opportunities often limited to the scope of the broadcaster, media provider or independent sports production company. Typically, people work at a job for some time before receiving a formal promotion. On the other hand promotions are often made internally.

Recent changes to workflows combined with substantially increased demand for sports content, means there have been more opportunities to enter sports television with many starting at assistant producer level. Promotion to producer can be faster but is often made within a limited terrain, i.e. working on a particular series or on a specific sport. For example, a junior assistant producer may find opportunities for progression within, say, Premier League Productions but, having progressed, might find it hard to transfer these skills to another sport. As Tunstall (1993:74) found, it is generally difficult for sports producers to export their skillset to other genres outside sport – in my experience this remains the case.

When television industry practices, including implementing short term contracts for production staff (including project-specific contracts), are aligned to a tendency towards annual programming commissions (even when rights are held for longer periods by broadcasters, annual production contracts are still often preferred) then the appearance of tram lines that can dictate career development is hardly a surprise. Increased demand for content is frequently offset by the constant pressure to reduce costs, including overheads and production fees, so with tighter production conditions this, again, reinforces the tendency to opt for more defined roles and appointing people with a reputation for delivering; for *replication* rather than *innovation*.

For some sports there are circumstantial reasons for specialisation, as the senior managers and producers interviewed in 2012 and 2013 confirmed. For example, a senior director with direct experience points out that directing Formula 1 coverage requires control of 50 or more cameras across a race circuit, there are additional in-car camera feeds, a vast array of replay options plus streams of performance-related data to process and present. An executive producer with broadcaster experience adds multi-sport coverage, as is the case with athletics, presents location and timing issues as events happen concurrently across the venue (the ability to stack EVS clips to give the impression of a constant flow of action and to offer some sort of narrative form is a specific skill). A specialist golf executive producer interviewed in 2012 confirmed that a similar technique is used where the broadcast action is usually a constantly updated flow of short clips from EVS. Sports including golf and world rally also require cameras to be rapidly relocated from one position to another to capture the action – this is another type of specialised directing that places a greater emphasis on logistics to provide effective coverage. For sports like football, rugby, cricket and tennis, producers and directors stressed the need to capture the rhythm and pace of each match, with replays and statistics added to assist commentary. Another senior producer pointed out that American sports, with their frequent breaks, offer further challenges that are met by deploying EVS and introducing a delay of up to three minutes from the incoming live feed to the outgoing broadcast presentation. Reviewing interviews with managers, producers and directors, overall there was a strong feeling that specialisation was a significant factor.

Speaking to producers and directors who are over 45 years old, their experiences are remarkably similar; many see themselves as 'the last of a dying breed' of multisport producers. For most of these producers their early experience was gained at a traditional broadcaster, like the BBC in the late 1980s and early 1990s where they worked on numerous sports. The managing director of a major independent sports production company echoed the senior manager that had worked on more than 40 different sports:

> There won't be any one else like me in the future, someone who has worked on everything. In every field, new projects [now] require specialists. (Managing director, independent sports production, 2012)

Whilst all the contributors interviewed felt sports production had entered an era of specialisation, there was less clarity about when this changed. In the 1990s and into the early 2000s, I wrote successful production service tenders for NBA (Channel Four and ITV), Rugby Special (BBC), Formula 1 (ITV) and World Rally Championships (Federation-based production). I can confirm it was still possible to offer 'a fresh pair of eyes' when designing coverage of sport for a broadcaster or even a federation. But, from around 2005 the scope for different ideas and new approaches appears to have narrowed significantly. In part, this is due to the rapid extension of Olympic Broadcasting Services and Host Broadcast Services, plus the expanded output of league-based operations like Premier League Productions; these commissioners prefer to use production specialists.

Broadcasters increasingly prefer production experts who know the unwritten rules when covering specific sports and that will not cause embarrassment with the league or federation from which the broadcaster has bought the rights. In the case of Channel Four horse racing, in 2012 IMG hired an executive producer from BBC Sport to deliver this expertise. With producers and directors providing the same expertise for different broadcasters, differences are likely to diminish further. Considering other reasons that could be driving specialisation, a senior series producer adds a useful perspective:

> There are so many new channels to fill. Before this [changed], you would work on six or seven sports in a year. But there is so much sport that needs to be filled you have to specialise in football, cricket, golf, snooker, darts and so on. Producers concentrate on that one sport to the exclusion of everything else. The transformation in the

volume of sport broadcast is responsible for specialisation. (Senior series producer, independent sports production, 2012)

This straightforward view has its merits. A full-service football channel broadcasting 24 hours a day, seven days a week will promote specialisation in football. But linking key producers and directors to coverage of specific sports is not new. Since the late 1980s, as independent sports production companies responded to production tenders, it was common practice to name individual senior producers or directors in the production contract for the duration of the series. Broadcasters were the first to do this but federations, too, became increasingly aware of the value specific producers and directors could add to their coverage. For example, ITV's Mike Watts was a favourite director of UEFA on Champions League coverage. Karl Hicks specialised in horse racing at the BBC and brought this experience via IMG Sports Media to Channel Four when, in 2012, the broadcaster acquired the rights to all significant racing in the UK. For many years Keith MacMillan was known for Formula 1 coverage at the BBC, when coverage moved to ITV in the mid-1990s MacMillan, now freelance, took charge of directing the British Grand Prix. Occasionally a director who has gained recognition in covering one sport, say Martin Turner who developed rugby union coverage at Sky Sports, will be used to help secure another contract, as was the case when Sky Sports acquired the majority of rights to broadcast Formula 1. From the mid-1990s federations were becoming more aware and more influential about which producers and directors would be acceptable to take charge of coverage.

What is new today is the intense pressure to specialise exerted by broadcasters and federations. As noted, for any tender response specialist knowledge is essential: 'Independents have to pitch with experts otherwise you won't get in', confirmed a senior executive producer speaking in 2013. This pressure is not exclusive to broadcasters: I recall the NBA tried to influence Channel Four in the choice of a sympathetic producer when Channel Four renewed its broadcasting rights for the NBA in the mid-1990s (the NBA had been wary of the editorial tone and choice of on-screen talent but, later, adopted these techniques and hired the talent directly). Similarly, in late 2013, when IMG Sports Media appointed a new executive producer to run Premier League Productions, it is reasonable to assume that approval from the Premier League was sought.

There is a further trend towards specialism that has had a direct influence on the day-to-day work of sports producers and directors, the rise of the production management department.

7.5 The rise of production management

Since the mid-1990s a new specialisation has emerged that mirrors the increasingly business-oriented aspects of television sports production: production management. A senior manager from a leading independent sports producer with a broadcaster background explains:

> Production managers and directors of production are very much an independent sports production thing. There were no such roles at the BBC, even now [there aren't any]. When independent sports production companies started they probably had producers who didn't have the experience of budgets that broadcasters had. (Senior manager, independent sports production, 2013)

My experience is that independent producers can deliver accurate budgets. Whilst not initially adopted at the BBC, production managers were certainly used in ITV sports departments from the early 1990s, with some then moving into independent production. But the most interesting link is between rise of production management and the increasing centrality of contracts, IP rights and the attachment of financial value to all stages of the television sports production chain as the sector has become more business-oriented.

Collating experience of working at several different independent producers, a typical pyramid structure in a production management department includes a director of production and several heads of production that oversee groups of productions. Roles usually assigned to a primary production include production executives, production managers, production co-ordinators and production secretaries. Among key responsibilities are: project budgeting, cost reporting (reconciling forecast budgets with actual spending), insurance, risk assessment, health and safety, scheduling (from travel and crewing to post production facilities), delivery, and all contract management (including engaging and authorising payments to freelance staff, plus the acquisition of any third party material and music usage reports). Issues to do with production quotas and Transfer of Undertakings (TUPE) may also arise but would involve liaison with senior managers and specialist lawyers. Whilst not a legal or business role *per se*, the striking growth in production management appears to reflect the ways in which previously informal relationships have come to be increasingly expressed through contracts and how financial values have become the determining factors of many more activities (Harvey, 2005). For example, all programme contributors should sign a consent/release form before interviews can be used. But the relatively simple task of acquiring a release form has become more complex due to (a) the increasingly legal expressions used, (b) the extent of the rights sought (often for all media in perpetuity), and (c) the token compensation offered for these rights by the production company (i.e., a fee of £1 is required to validate the agreement). This has made the process more complicated and invites interrogation from contributors' agents who are likely to attach a much higher value to the contribution as they anticipate it will be recycled (and monetised) in numerous alternative forms.

In contrast to the group of special advisors to leagues and federations dominated by men, women fulfil the majority of roles in production management. At IMG Sports Media – apart from the director of production and a single head of production – the department (including five further heads of production and numerous production managers and co-ordinators) features female staff. There are almost no female producers.

Another revealing division can be seen in the terms used to engage staff. Whilst the majority of more senior production managers are offered staff contracts within the independent sports production sector the trend is towards issuing short-term contracts to all producers, directors and assistant producers. Speaking in 2013 IMG's director of production confirmed the company was 'moving towards a contract-based' policy with contracts tied to specific productions. This ensures full recovery of all costs, particularly salaries (for example, by limiting engagement to a single season of UEFA Champions League magazine shows, including a mid-season two month unpaid break). Once the over-arching production contract expires (i.e., the contract between the commissioner and the independent sports production company) the expectation is that production staff will be released unless other projects are available. With senior production managers on staff terms and producers, directors and assistant producers increasingly employed on short-term project-specific contracts, whether intentional or not a divisive power imbalance exists.

As production management has extended its influence in television sports production, many of the duties once carried out by senior and executive producers – for example, budgeting – have been curtailed, with producers now encouraged to focus on creative and editorial input rather than contracts and costs. One executive producer in charge of a prominent weekly magazine show at an independent sports production company speaking in 2012 confirmed he 'had no idea about the programme budget'. 'I don't pay much attention to that', he added, even though his production was running over budget and causing alarm. In addition to gaps in information, a senior executive producer now working in independent sports production explains some tensions in play:

> I was used to a team including a producer, a production assistant and a technical manager. That's it. The production manager role was new to me; I'm still not 100% clear what his or her role is. At first it seems more financial, but then they'll get involved in booking a satellite ... Heads of Production definitely try it on with younger producers because they can, but not with old and haggard producers like me. (Senior executive producer, independent sports production, 2013)

Many producers interviewed confided they were happy to work with production managers, but most found the role of head of production more vexing as questions of authority arose – who is in charge? In 2011 I was executive producer of a new series of documentaries made by IMG Sports Media. Formally introducing the IMG team to the client it was made clear, by the director of production, that the team leader was the head of production. The head of production was a member of staff, the executive producer role was on short-term contract. Examples like this signal the central importance of contracts and compliance in day-to-day production matters.

Among the younger producers interviewed, many viewed production management as acting as some sort of internal policing, constraining programme spending, enforcing compliance and various contractual activities, ranging from the use of third-party footage and music to risk assessments and insurance reports.

The tension continues as production managers frequently view producers as being undisciplined or lacking motivation when it comes to meeting assigned budgets and carrying out necessary administrative duties, including providing signed consent forms, clearing third party content and declaring music usage in completed programmes. As one senior production executive confirmed:

> I am sick of playing the bad cop, chasing up clearances and contributor release forms that producers can't be bothered to get signed when they are shooting, but know they should have done. We go to great lengths to let them [producers] know exactly what they need

to do, but when they don't even bother to read the guidelines they are given it becomes very frustrating. (Senior production executive, independent sports production, 2012.)

These comments, made by a respected production executive at a leading independent sports production company, represent a typical response. Many production managers working in sport revealed they felt undervalued by the producers they work with and some felt undervalued by the company. The split between editorial and operational management is an important trend that, intentionally or not, sees producers and directors being led away from the business-side of production. As they also see opportunities for creative input reduced – particularly in respect of league and federation run productions – then friction cannot come as a surprise. In some respects this situation can be regarded a consequence of the rapid expansion of the downstream content provision market and the financialisation of independent sports production activities.

Regulations and approvals

Briefly returning to media regulation, regional production quotas and Transfer of Undertakings (TUPE), it is reasonable to conclude that company managers, heads of production and executive producers have primary interaction with these areas, with most producers happy to keep such matters at arm's length. However, the rise of health and safety and third party liability usually has a more direct impact on production. An experienced director working on live international productions explains the changes he has noticed:

Health and safety is the biggest element in live production. Cables laid near athletes or the public and working at heights are a no go compared to 15 years ago. There is a lot more preparation – and health and safety in place – to get Bob up on a wall so you can get your nice wide shot. But, increasingly, there are also cultural considerations. For example, how women are expected to dress when working in the Middle-East. (Live international sports director, 2012)

Television sport is not the only industry to see health and safety management spread. In any case, as the scale of outside broadcast and major event coverage has increased markedly they have attracted more scrutiny. Most independent sports production companies run health and safety courses that require staff to update their understanding on a regular basis. However, issues to do with conduct and security are relatively new developments. A film about the Anzi Makhachkala football team based in Dagestan (an unstable federal republic of Russia located in the North Caucasus by the Caspian Sea) that I supervised for IMG in 2011 required a detailed specialist security report to be carried out and recommendations for safety set out before the production could proceed. Similar conditions apply for sports events held on remote or in potentially dangerous locations, this includes the last two World Cup Finals in South Africa and Brazil.

Discussing the changing demands of the role prompted contributing producers to raise a further concern: the increasing layers of editorial approval now required, both internal and external, compared to 15 years ago.

Whether it is (a) a broadcaster's commissioning executives, genre heads and channel controller, (b) intervention directly from leagues or sponsors, or (c) production manuals prepared by federations, the perception is there are far more steps spanning a wider range of editorial decisions. To some extent this may be a hangover as sports producers adjust to the reality of working for different clients and that, in the past, they had enjoyed significant freedom during live broadcasts where direct intervention is less practical. Further levels of supervision also reflect the increased importance of sports content to rights-holding broadcasters.

Two examples from Channel Four illustrate the extent of change. In 1998 I produced the first series of *Sumo*. Although none of the content had been viewed, Channel Four arranged a large press/publicity screening. Just before the screening began, Adrian Metcalf, the commissioning editor, quietly called me over. 'Mike, the programmes are okay, aren't they?' Fortunately they were well received. Spooling forward to 2012 and as relayed in 2013 by a senior producer who was present throughout, Channel Four convened a press conference to announce the line-up of presenters for their 2012 Paralympic coverage. The commissioning editor and production teams had worked for some time to compile these teams, including screen testing them on various Channel Four programmes. Following the press launch Channel Four's chief creative officer, Jay Hunt, unilaterally decided to make wholesale changes to the line-ups. This case illustrates the underlying importance of sports presentation to a channel, plus how an increase in the number of editorial decision makers in the programme production chain tends to diminish the influence of the producer.

Conclusion

Chapter 7 examined how pre-production processes impact on independent sports television production, from company-level activities to the shop floor and the day-to-day work of sports producers and directors. A micro-level view was added to the supply side perspective provided throughout this book; a gap in describing the contemporary television sport production environment was also filled. Reasons why transformations in television sports production have not resulted in a creative heyday for sports producers and directors were reviewed and, instead, it was noted that inhibition and prescription have become recurring themes.

The chapter opened with an introduction to the UK independent sports production sector. Independent sport production companies face several significant challenges: 1) they do not usually hold any sports broadcasting rights, 2) they do not have direct access to audiences, 3) operations are usually on a small scale, 4) companies are increasingly controlled by private equity firms or are part of larger independent media groups, and 5) the cyclical nature of sports rights means winning competitive tenders for production services is a vital and costly activity.

The commissioning process for independent sports production services was reviewed. As they seldom hold rights (even secondary rights) independent sports production companies sell their production services at costs plus a percentage fee primarily to broadcasters but, increasingly, directly to leagues and federations as these organisations extend their own production operations. The different demands made by content commissioners were discussed. In important ways these demands can be considered just as influential as technology in shaping the final output we see.

A number of factors, including a substantial increase in demand for content and the prominence of live sports broadcasting (with its increased technical and logistical complexity), when added to the limited scope of output offered by most independent sports production companies has created considerable pressure to specialise in the sports that they cover. The question of whether *replication* had become more important than *originality* was raised. The tension experienced between (a) providing a more standardised international coverage for federations, or (b) more localised presentation for broadcasters was discussed. It was argued that the introduction of standardised and approved coverage by federations is a new kind of content – a new media-sports product – and another important step in the commodification of television sport. As sports television is increasingly assimilated within the growing marketisation and promotional culture of sport, independent sports production companies, producers and directors have to *play by the rules, or not play at all*. This condition is one of the most fundamental changes to television sport production in the past decade.

The chapter concluded by identifying further specialisation in television sports production: the emergence of production management. Marked divisions between editorial and operational management in downstream content provision were discussed including the tensions felt on both sides, by producers and production managers. The tendency for senior production management roles to benefit from staff positions, whilst producers and directors are increasingly engaged on short-term project-specific contracts was identified and a further power shift away from producers was noted. How increasing layers of approval that producers are required to navigate through was provided in two examples from Channel Four. Overall, sports producers said they felt their role was diminishing.

8
Conclusion

This book has argued that the transformation of television sport has been driven by a combination of interacting forces including technology, broadcasting rights (economics) and media regulation (politics). These forces mostly operate upstream and out of sight (i.e. before traditional production and distribution processes begin) and increasingly determine what sport we see where we can see and what the final output looks and sounds like.

Two critical perspectives currently missing from political economy accounts were identified and added: 1) the central role of sports federations, from the application of sports economics to federation-run host broadcast coverage and branded channel provision, and 2) a relevant analysis of supply-side activities that map the impact of pre-production transformations. The book set out to provide a view that complements existing demand side political economy interpretations and offers a convincing explanation of how television sports programmes are made, who makes them and why programmes look and sound as they do.

The battle to control broadcasting rights and subsequent television output was viewed against the increasing commercialisation of sport and the marketisation of broadcasting. The speed and scale of transformation has been remarkable and many of the outcomes have yet to receive scrutiny, including:

• The expansion of federation-based production activities. This includes host broadcast production (providing sympathetic coverage for global audiences) and branded-content channels with extensive international distribution.
• An increase in detailed production prescriptions required of rights-holding broadcasters as a key part of broadcasting rights agreements.

- As organising federation provide international *coverage* of major sports how broadcasters increasingly concentrate on *presentation* (as approved global feeds are localised and re-branded by broadcasters for their domestic audience).
- The pressure on independent sports production companies, including producers and directors, to offer increasingly specialised production services.
- The ultimate requirement: that all television sport production companies, producers and directors *play by the rules or don't play at all*.

The arrival of digital technology in the mid-1990s accelerated and intensified these processes. Mason (1999:403) argues that sport has commodified as it has become increasingly bound up in the processes of economic production and distribution. Looking at sport as a media product, it can be argued that intellectual property rights have been used to 'inhibit rather than encourage creation and creativity' (Haynes, 2005:10) and, overall, there is a 'danger based on the quiet accretion of restrictions' (Drahos and Braithwaite, 2002:4). Viewed against the rising tide of neoliberal values – where the neoliberal project involving the 'financialisation of everything' (Harvey, 2005:33) and 'accumulation through dispossession' (Harvey, 2005:159) is apparent – then commercial values and the market are the driving forces in the digital era of television sport.

Today, the Premier League demonstrates unprecedented levels of corporate organisation and profit-driven motivation, even surpassing some of the activities of the NFL, a league that has set the benchmark for commercial activity since the 1970s. This transformation was driven by a trinity of technological, economic, and political forces that combined in various ways to create a world where what is good for business is considered to be good for us all (Harvey, 2005:117). Understanding this transformation requires engaging with league and federation behaviour. There are seven developments of note:

1) The NFL was the first professional sports league to understand the importance of (a) the collective sale of sports broadcasting rights (cartel behaviour), (b) providing league-wide sporting equilibrium (competitive balance and uncertainty of outcome), and (c) exercising its market power to collect this value. With scarcity came rationing, as there was no effective substitute for the NFL it became a seller's market. The price of NFL rights rose steadily from the 1970s.

2) The formalisation of global corporate sponsorship as a viable alternative to advertising in the 1980s was a critical development that had a profound impact on the growth of global sports events, including the Olympics and the World Cup Finals. The amalgamation of sport, television and corporate interests into a *single package* was commercially successful and, from the landmark 1984 Los Angeles Games, the IOC moved forward on a more aggressively commercial basis as it sought ways to deliver a television product that was entirely sympathetic to the requirements of its preferred sponsors (The Olympic Programme, TOP). Similarly, FIFA increased its revenues from advertising, sponsorship and broadcasting rights from the early 1980s, with the biggest gains coming from 1986 onwards.

3) In the late 1980s the NBA overtly allied its sport media product to entertainment values and celebrity endorsements that, together, helped to create (a) a global NBA brand that was exported worldwide, and (b) to propel the increasingly commercial culture of modern sport into the mainstream.

4) Marketing activities also changed federations' view of audiences. In the 1980s and 1990s, as it sold its broadcasting rights into more international markets, Formula 1 began to focus on global rather than local audiences. F1 actively sought a consistent television output across an entire season, moving from race to race and country to country. Although Formula 1 could not make a commercial success of its own pay-TV coverage, it did begin to re-define television/sport relationships, particularly where federations would play an increasingly significant role in identifying and delivering standardised coverage of their own events for global audiences. F1 was also at the vanguard of identifying increasingly specific conditions under which its events could be broadcast.

5) Under acute commercial pressure from Europe's leading clubs, the UEFA Champions League was launched in 1992. Working with TEAM Marketing AG, many of the lessons learned by the IOC, FIFA and Formula 1 were re-articulated. As a formal obligation, UEFA required all rights-holding broadcasters to comply with the prescriptions set out in its Production Manual. The UEFA Champions League Production Manual set a new benchmark when attaching conditions to sports broadcasting rights and imposing these requirements on broadcasters' output.

6) The creation of the Premier League in 1992 signaled the most rational approach to capital accumulation so far by any British sport. With its corporate structure and commercial autonomy, the Premier League is driven by an unambiguous profit motive. In some

important ways it can be argued that the Premier League has become even more commercial and profit-driven than the NFL, both in terms of its structure, where members act as shareholders, and with the increasing revenues for broadcasting rights it has achieved globally.
7) The emergence, around 2005, of federation-run host broadcast operations at major sports events is very significant. Approved and non-controversial coverage for global audiences was now delivered to all rights-holding broadcasters.

Chapter 2 filled in a missing back-story with a comparison of the development of sport and television in the US and UK between 1945 and 1995. Starting from virtually opposite positions post-World War II, and as 'the rule of amateurs kept capitalism at bay in British sport' (Holt, 1989:281), sport in the UK was poised between an idealised past and a commercialised free-market future. This proved to be a mismatch. As sport disengaged from the wider social and cultural meanings that had kept it firmly anchored, in the race between money and meaning there was only ever likely to be one winner. When the tide turned, in the 1980s, it did so quickly and sport and television became realigned along commercial and consumer-oriented structures more typically seen in the US.

By the mid-1990s, elite sport had come to matter a great deal to big business and to managers of increasingly commercial and global media industries. 'Sports now stress the need to be business-like and efficient, offer sites for the celebration of corporate capitalism ... and, in general have become prime sites for the construction and reproduction of an entrepreneurial culture', concluded Whannel (1992:208). For the media industries, Boyle and Haynes (2000:222) added, sport 'offers a product, which can be transformed into a valuable commercial entity delivering readers, viewers, advertisers, customers and subscribers. Sport, it appears, is often only too happy to oblige as a willing victim in this process'. Following this trajectory, Falcous (2005) found that professional sport had become realigned with the interests of corporate investment and the managerial tenets of advertising, marketing and public relations. A new sport-media-corporate axis had emerged.

Across the next three chapters, how a trinity of influential pre-production factors, technology, broadcasting rights (economics) and regulation (politics) have been instrumental in transforming television sport since the early 1990s was examined.

Chapter 3 focussed on technology. On the supply side, the increasing prominence of live sports broadcasting, driven by the arrival of Sky Sports in 1992, was not based on new technology so much as on using more of the existing technology in new ways. Via encrypted satellite transmission, a solution to market failure was found by charging customers monthly subscriptions to access encoded signals, as popular sports became *private goods*, hidden from general access behind a pay wall. For Boyle and Haynes (2004:20), this marked the transformation of viewers from citizens to consumers. Aligned to an aggressive marketing strategy, Sky Sports adopted several overtly US methods and continued Roone Arledge's close up and personal philosophy. Rising to levels of importance found in the US, *live* sports broadcasting soon became the definitive form for television sport in the UK.

Although transmission operations at broadcasting networks were among the first areas to adopt automated digital systems, the transition to a fully digital and tape-free workflow was not straightforward. A lack of common standards remains problematic. By contrast, the arrival of new methods and much faster ways of working, dovetailed perfectly into a reconfigured television sports environment; potential output was radically transformed. Whilst large volumes of media could be transferred between locations, it was the capability to allow *simultaneous* access by *numerous* clients to the same *original material* that was revolutionary. Two important phases can be noted: 1) between 1994 and 2004 key non-linear editing and tapeless media technology was rolled out; introduced to production workflows this technology enabled a greatly increased volume and scope of sports content to be produced much faster than ever before, and 2) from 2004 onwards, how sports federations, including the Premier League, were able to harness this potential to produce, under their own control, a guaranteed standard for global output that was closely aligned to their own brand values. In this case it is not the technology itself, but *who* uses the technology and *why* that is revealing. The mid-2000s saw federations move the goalposts further as they took charge of their own television coverage at major sports events.

The Premier League's production arm, Premier League Productions was considered. Reviewing new methods and massively increased output illustrated how a *single minute* of live football action is transformed into *11 minutes* of programming designed for worldwide consumption delivered via a dedicated channel offering 168 hours of Premier League content each week. Operating at an entirely new level of commodification, Premier League Production's digital output represents a quantum leap from the BBC's 1992 analogue-based *Match of The Day* operation.

In contrast to fast moving developments in technology, including the capacity to create more content, more quickly for use on more platforms, any discussion of broadcasting rights tends to involve a rapid deceleration; rights are usually about what you *cannot* do. How leagues and federations have engaged in cartel behaviour to gain market power was explained, including how the use of prescriptive conditions (added to broadcasting rights by league and federations) reinforces their dominant position. These are critical developments.

Chapter 4 reviewed the nature of intellectual property, including (a) how intellectual property knows no bounds (Haynes, 2005), (b) the confusing idea/expression dichotomy, and (c) the tendency of copyright to be defined by market-driven principles that demarcate who owns what. Without a homogenised approach to international copyright, individual states sanction and regulate intellectual property rights. The utilitarian, market-driven principles of copyright (and how they are interpreted by contemporary global media companies) have increasingly become the *de facto* understanding of how media rights are valued, organised and distributed. In terms of sports broadcasting rights in the UK, values began to escalate from the late 1980s. Using the Premier League as an example, factors that shape value were explained and the different ways that rights are broken down (by range, distribution platform, broadcast territory and period of license) were discussed, including the revenues achieved for Premier League broadcasting rights. As the cost of sports broadcasting rights escalate to record levels, a corresponding increase in the risks associated with acquiring such rights was identified, including the consequences of over valuing or losing important rights.

Among concerns raised in the application of intellectual property rights is what Drahos and Braithwaite (2002) describe as a 'quiet accretion of restrictions', or what Harvey (2005:159) has, in more general terms, called 'accumulation though dispossession'. For television sport, these are largely unseen activities manifest in prescriptions that are applied to production. How leagues and federations have exercised their market power through typical prescriptions was illustrated with two case studies from Formula 1 and the UEFA Champions League.

The third pre-production factor that influences what sport we can see on television, including who makes the final programmes, is regulation – the focus of Chapter 5. If broadcasting rights can be considered to follow one cycle (typically three years) behind developments in technology, then regulators and competition authorities in the EU and UK often follow a further step behind. For Boyle and Haynes (2004:52) 'a re-regulation of broadcasting is taking place within a more commercial and market-driven frame of reference'.

Attitudes towards regulation differ in the US, UK and Europe. For Jeanrenaud and Kesenne (2006) sport in the US is seen as a commodity that can be redesigned as required, whereas in Europe sport is considered part of the cultural heritage; sport cannot be reduced to an audience-generating mechanism alone. Following deregulation in the UK, market forces increasingly determined broadcasting markets.

For sports broadcasting rights, intervention involves (a) listed events legislation (first adopted in the UK in 1954 and the EC from 1996), and (b) the application of competition law to correct market failure and address the market power of dominant pay-TV broadcasters. It was EC intervention that finally ended BSkyB's monopoly hold on exclusive Premier League broadcasting rights in 2005. Whilst the Premier League realised a significant escalation in the value it receives for rights, the cost to consumers who wanted to watch Premier League football increased. These were unlikely to be the outcomes sought by intervention. Lying outside the protected list of events the activities of the Premier league and UEFA have attracted considerable scrutiny.

Even within literature on regulation and competition, the picture remains frustratingly incomplete. From the programme supply side there are further dimensions that should be considered, including: 1) important areas not covered by regulators and competition author-ities (including the activities of leagues and federations as they provide coverage for major sporting events, or running international channels), and 2) the effects of regulation that impacts *directly* on production, following (a) the regulation of content, (b) regional and independent production quotas, and (c) recent EU employment legislation such as Transfer of Undertakings (TUPE) – these issues were described by contrib-utors as having a 'massive impact' on independent sports production.

Two examples from the US were considered relevant in finding a solu-tion. The US leagues have adopted voluntary forms of self-regulation and, whilst this is not the case in the UK, this may be a useful area to explore in the future, particularly as UEFA introduced Financial Fair Play rules for the 2013–14 season. Even without a list of protected events, the US Major Leagues have not migrated to pay-TV but, instead, have main-tained a strong presence on the four commercial free-to-air networks. Although the US market is much larger than the UK and the owner-ship of rights to all four major leagues by any one broadcaster is, for cost reasons alone, highly unlikely, in general terms Evens, Iosifidis and Smith (2013:228) conclude the increased exposure and higher audience ratings via free-to-air television in the US example *can* serve the interest of teams, leagues, broadcasters, advertisers, sponsors and viewers alike.

It was concluded that there are troubling gaps between the poten-tially valuable underlying intentions of intervention and the practical outcomes delivered. As Boyle and Haynes (2004:165) put it: 'regulators strive to keep pace with a digital mediascape which threatens to perpetually run ahead of regulatory frameworks'. As moves by federations to take control of their own host broadcast coverage, and leagues to distribute their own global content, could leave regulators even further adrift, it was argued there was a need for new ways of thinking about regulation, including looking at (a) the solutions adopted by the US leagues, and (b) how leagues and federations might consider the example set by the German Bundesliga, where the game is considered to be a *public good* and where football, not the exclusive pursuit of financial revenues, remains at the heart of all club activities.

Chapters 6 and 7 provided a micro-level analysis of the contemporary supply-side in television sport, including challenges faced by broadcasters and independent sports production as the effects of transformations in technology, broadcasting rights and regulation trickle down to the workplace. For broadcasters the challenges include: (a) the increasingly close relationship between sports broadcasting rights ownership and the commercial performance of large media firms (for example BT Sport and BSkyB), (b) the consequences of federation-based host broadcast coverage for major events and how, (c) this has created a division between event *coverage* designed for global audiences and *presentation* for local audiences increasingly offered by broadcasters. Additionally, (d) how increased demand for sports content has failed to deliver any meaningful critical comment was noted; for Boyle and Haynes (2000:107) television knows 'that it must not kill the goose that lays the golden eggs'.

In an oligopolistic market structure, changes in sports broadcasting rights ownership directly impact on the economic performance of competing companies; the growing significance of corporate performance suggests the way in which sports broadcasting rights are valued is becoming more complex. As the escalation in prices paid for sports broadcasting rights show no sign of slowing, the possibility of encountering *winners curse* increases; of bidding too much for rights. An interesting scenario could play out if, sensing a commercial opportunity, a very large company like Google or Microsoft were to enter the market for broadcasting rights and potentially change the viewing paradigm – this view concurs with Evens, Iosifidis and Smith (2013). The move by Discovery in 2015 to secure pan-European rights for the Olympics illustrates how one firm's action can have widespread impact.

The emergence of federation-run production operations is one of the most significant developments in television sport as it changes the rules of engagement with broadcasters and producers; in a sense an intermediary level of production has been removed. The IOC, FIFA and UEFA now seek control of *every aspect of production* as they provide a dependable and sympathetic international feed of coverage to all rights holding broadcasters. In doing so, the line between what is best for advertisers/sponsors and broadcasters becomes increasingly blurred. Gruneau and Cantelon (1988:347) note how the Olympics have become a market-oriented project where 'a more fully developed expression of incorporation of sporting practice into the ever-expanding marketplace of international capitalism is now manifested'. Federation-based production is a *critical new phase* in television sports production, one that illustrates the extent that power has migrated to the leagues and federations.

As broadcasters respond to federation-run broadcast coverage, and by buying in further coverage from other broadcasters to fill expanding television sports schedules, then the importance of *presentation* as a distinct aspect of production activity has increased significantly since 2005. Whilst the BBC is frequently beaten in commercial competition to acquire sports broadcasting rights, the corporation still has access to the Olympics (until 2018), World Cup Finals and Euro Championships. As coverage of major international sports events is provided by the federations this has released the BBC to concentrate its efforts and resources on the presentation of major events. Presentation is the shoulder programming that wraps around the provided international coverage and that, importantly, the BBC localises for UK viewers. Presentation is also a means to differentiate broadcast output and to build a recognisable brand identity. Despite losing many key rights, the BBC has retained a plausible position as the broadcaster that can deliver a shared viewing experience for large numbers of British viewers. Presentation is one of the remaining areas where broadcasters still retain substantial control, so is of particular interest.

Why transformations in television sport did not provide a foundation for a creative heyday for sports producers and directors but has 'inhibited innovation and creativity' (Haynes, 2005:10) was addressed in Chapter 7 and the day-to-day work of independent sports production companies. Independent sports production companies face several challenges: 1) they do not hold sports broadcasting rights, 2) they do not have direct access to audiences, 3) operation is often on a relatively small scale, 4) companies are increasingly controlled by private equity firms seeking short-term returns, or are part of larger independent media groups, and 5) the cyclical nature of sports rights means that winning competition tenders to provide production services is a critical concern.

Given their already limited scope, these factors encourage independent sports production companies to specialise.

Unlike other areas of independent production, sports production companies tend not to hold secondary rights so they sell their services at costs plus a percentage production fee. Their primary customers are broadcasters but, increasingly, leagues and federations also seek short-term production expertise to support their host broadcast operations. The different demands of federations (reaching a global audience, non-controversial output, often very prescriptive) and broadcasters (local audiences, increasingly focussed on presentation rather than coverage, occasionally more creative) are significant and, in several important ways, these demands are extremely influential in shaping the final output.

A number of other factors, including (a) substantial increase in demand for sports content and (b) the prominence of live sports broadcasting (including technical complexity and logistics) when added to (c) the limited scope of output usually offered by independent sports production companies, generates further specialisation. This raises questions including whether *replication* is now more important than *originality* in television sports. As sports television is increasingly assimilated within the growing marketisation and promotional culture of sport, it was argued that broadcasters, independent sports production companies, producers and directors now have to play by the federations' rules. This is one of the most fundamental and important changes to television sport since 2005.

Further evidence of specialisation is found in the emergence of production management. Over the past decade, a marked division between *editorial* and *operational* management in television sports content provision is evident. The tendency for senior production management roles to occupy a limited number of core staff positions at independent sports production companies, whilst producers and directors are increasingly engaged on short-term project-specific contracts indicates the role of sports producer is, in general terms, diminishing. Whether a result of adjusting to the needs of having more clients, the growing importance of sports rights to broadcasters or simply the centrality of broadcasters presentation strategy, virtually all producers interviewed noted they were required to navigate through more levels of supervision and approval than in the past. The universal message from sports producers and directors was that of increasing specialisation and prescription in their work, with less and less room afforded for creativity. Describing what it is like to work for a federation, memorably one producer said: 'the difference is like living in a democracy and living in

North Korea'. Even allowing for some exaggeration, the differences are not subtle.

The paradox of television sports production

Boyle and Haynes (2000:38) wrote: 'a history of sport is often presented as a history of televising sport'. On the subject of television sport they add: 'what is significant is the scale and the intensity that now exists within this relationship and the rapid pace of change which characterises the media and sporting industries' (2000:x, preface). Today, the intensity and pace of change has accelerated to unprecedented levels as the leagues and federations that run sport have become increasingly powerful.

Following the landmark 1990 Broadcasting Act, 1992 was a pivotal year in the transformation of television sport in the UK – BSkyB launched with live and exclusive coverage of the newly formed Premier League and the UEFA Champions League format was rolled out with its Production Manuals and embedded sponsorship model. The mid-2000s provided another critical turning point as new digital technology, intellectual property control and lack of applicable media regulations allowed leagues and federations to seize even more control of television sport through host-broadcast operations and providing their own brand-name sport channels for widespread international distribution. In the early 1990s Tunstall (1993:72) was concerned that the prominence placed on technology and logistics in television sport could diminish the journalistic value of the content. What journalistic value that remains appears to have migrated from standardised international *coverage* designed for global audiences to the *presentation* offered by rights holding broadcasters as they repackage and brand events for local audiences.

Having worked through this period, it is my view that television sport has entered a particularly paradoxical phase. On one hand the technical capacity and specialist production skills deployed in capturing and conveying elite sports performance on television, particularly in the UK, US and at major global events, can produce breath-taking coverage; incredibly detailed sequences and atmospheric audio that combine in unforgettable programmes showcasing a wide range of human performance, drama and emotion. At its best, television sport can be captivating, compelling and memorable. On the other hand, even the most outstanding coverage can quickly become one-dimensional as it seeks to avoid all controversy and provide the most sympathetic and uncritical coverage on behalf of the host federation and its key commercial partners. Whilst there have been enormous increases in the volume of sports television coverage, including more scope than ever before, the overall gravitational pull is towards generating more and more standardised global television sport products. It has become the role of rights-holding broadcasters, should they be motivated to do so, to localise this coverage via presentation defined by their editorial approach, style and on-screen talent. Above all, this is an era where criticism of leagues and federations is not encouraged – with so much money invested in winning and retaining popular sports broadcasting rights, or in winning production service contracts, who dares to bite the hand that feeds?

As Boyle and Haynes (2004:167) point out, sport has a remarkable ability to re-invent itself as new technology has come along. Similarly, the battle to control sport is not new, although, it is argued here, that the battle has entered a new and more intense phase where the leagues and federations have become even more dominant. Today's extremely sophisticated television sports coverage, drawing on an unprecedented arsenal of digital technology, high-capacity workflows and battalions of ever-more specialised producers and directors, has one objective: to remain in thrall to sport. A political economy perspective asks if a working balance can be found between short-term gain and long-term wellbeing, between local and global priorities and, most of all, between making money and cultural/historical meaning? Until some checks and balances can be restored – and it was argued that these should come from the leagues and federations – then contemporary television sport will be ever more closely aligned to elite sport's wider global marketing objectives and profit targets. With FIFA and the IAAF under investigation for corruption, this is should be a concern.

Television sport has been totally transformed; the goalposts have moved and the rules have been changed. As it continues to attract mass audiences, there is little doubt that live coverage and subsequent presentation of elite sport sets new standards for scope and sophistication, for technical excellence. The appeal of television sport seems undiminished. However, in the same way that broadcasters are carried along on the bow wave of sport's commercial rapacity, whether they like it or not, whether they admit it or not, today's sports production companies, individual sport producers and directors are all part of this market-led momentum. The message is simple: you play by the new rules, or you don't play at all.

References

Andreff W and J Bourg (2006) 'Watching the Football Game: Broadcasting Rights for the European digital television Market', Journal of Sport and Social Issues, February 2011, 35: pp 33–49

Banks, S (2002) Going Down: Football in Crisis, Edinburgh & London: Mainstream

Barnett, S (1990) Games and Sets, The Changing Face of Sport on Television. London: BFI

BBC (2013) 'Champions League: BT wins £897 million football rights deal.' Available online at www.bbc.co.uk/sport/0/football/24879138 [Accessed 30 June 2015]

Booth, D and G Doyle (1997) 'UK TV warms up to the biggest game yet: Pay-Per-View', Media, Culture and Society, 19(2): pp 277–284

Boyle, R and R Haynes (2000) Power play: sport, the media and popular culture. London: Longman

Boyle, R and R Haynes (2004), Football in the New Media Age. London: Routledge

Brander, J and B Spencer (1983) 'International R + D Rivalry and Industrial Strategy', Review of Economic Studies, 50(4): pp 707–722

Briggs, S (2011) 'How Sky Sports became one of the most influential sports broadcasters over the last 20 years', The Telegraph, 18 April 2011

Brignall, M (2013) 'BT sorry for poor TV service after launch of sports channel', The Guardian 13 December 2013

Broadcasting Act 1990, London: HMSO. Available online at www.legislation.gov.uk/ukpga/1990/42/contents [Accessed 12 May 2014]

BSkyB (2013) BSkyB Group plc Annual Report 2013. Available online at www.corporate.sky.com/documents/pdf/publications/2013/annual_report_2013.pdf [Accessed 12 May 2014]

Burns, T (1977) The BBC: Public Institution and Private World, London: MacMillan

Calvin, M (2013) 'BT Sport wins rights to Champions League football: How TV's balance of power has been shifted by £879m deal that blows Sky Sports out of the water.' The Independent, 10 November 2013.

Cock, G (1930) Writing in the Radio Times, March 1930 and cited in Boyle and Haynes (2000) Power play: sport, the media and popular culture, London: Longman

Conn, D (1997) The Football Business: fair game in the '90s? Edinburgh: Mainstream

Considine, P (2013) 'North One to produce BT Sport MotoGP coverage', Television, 12 December 2013

Cook, C (2014) 'Channel 4 Racing defends record as 2013 figures show audience slump', The Guardian, 31 January 2014

Copyright Designs and Patent Act (1988) Available online at www.legislation.gov.uk/ukpga/1988/48/contents [Accessed 10 July 2015]

Copyright Related Rights Regulations (2003) Available online at http://www.legislation.gov.uk/uksi/2003/2498/made [Accessed 10 July 2015]

Cottle, S (ed) (2003) Media Organization and Production. London: Sage

Cowie C and M Williams (1997) *The Economics of Sports Rights*, Telecommunications Policy, 21(7), pp 619–34

Curran, J and J Seaton (2003) *Power without Responsibility. The press, broadcasting and new media in Britain*. London: Routledge

DCMS (2009) Available online at www.culture.gov.uk/freetoair/faq.html#17 [Accessed 30 July 2009]

Desbordes, M (2006) *Marketing and Football: An International Perspective*, Oxford: Butterworth-Heinemann

Dobson, S and J Goddard (2007) *The Economics of Football*, Cambridge: Cambridge University Press

Doyle, G (2002) *Understanding Media Economics*, London: Sage

Drahos, P and J Braithwaite (2002) *Information Feudalism, Who Owns the Knowledge Economy?* London: Earthscan

EC (1997) *Television without Frontiers and Major (Sports) Events: Commission Communications*. EC Press Release, 05 February 1997

Elstein, D (2010) *The Ofcom pay TV review: what does it really mean?* Opendemocracy.net 2 April 2010. Available online at www.opendemocracy.net/ourkingdom/david-elstein/ofcom-pay TV-review-what-does-it-really-mean [Accessed 22 October 2013]

Enders Analysis (2013) *BT Sport Euro football winner – what a price*, Nov 2013. Available online at www.endersanalysis.com/content/publication/bt-sport-euro-football-winner---what-price [Accessed 25 November 2013]

European Commission (1999) First European Conference on Sports, Olympia (Greece), 20–23 May

Evens, T, P Iosifidis and P Smith (2013) *The Political Economy of Television Sports Rights*. Basingstoke: Palgrave MacMillan

Falcous, M (2005) *'Global Struggles, Local Impacts: Rugby League, Rupert Murdoch's Global Vision and Cultural Identities'*, pp 57–84 in Nauright, J and K Schimmel (eds) (2005) The Political Economy of Sport. London: Palgrave MacMillan

Farrell, S (2015) *'Sky shares slide after Premier League TV rights deal'*, The Guardian, 11 February 2015.

Fernández Peña, E (2009) *'Olympic Summer Games and Broadcast Rights. Evolution and Challenges in the New Media Environment'*. Revista Latina de Comunicación Social, 64, pages 1.000 to 1.010. Laguna (Tenerife): Universidad de La Laguna

FIFA (2009) Available online at www.fifa.com/aboutfifa/index.html [Accessed 13 August 2009]

Fikentscher, A (2006) *'Joint Purchasing of Sports Rights: A Legal Viewpoint'*, in The Economics of Sport and the Media (2006). Cheltenham: Edward Elgar, pp 71–92

Forrest, D, R Simmons and B Buraimo (2006) *'Broadcaster and Audience Demand for Premier League Football'*, in Jeanrenaud C and S Kesenne (eds) (2006) The Economics of Sport and the Media. Cheltenham: Edward Elgar, pp 93–105

Fort, R (2006) *Sports Economics*, Upper Saddle River, New Jersey: Pearson

Fynn A and L Guest (1994) *Out of Time*. London: Simon & Schuster

Garside, J (2014) *'BT's push into football and fibre broadband drives up revenues'*, The Guardian, 31 January 2014

Garside, J (2015) *'BT Sport to charge for top-flight European football from August.'* The Guardian, 9 June 2015

Gerrard (2006) *'Competitive Balance and the Sports Media Rights Market: What are the Real Issues?'* in Jeanrenaud C, and S Kesenne (eds) (2006) The Economics of Sport and the Media. Cheltenham: Edward Elgar, pp 26–36

Gibson, O (2008) *'F1 returns to BBC but ITV wins Champions League.'* The Guardian, 21 March 2008

Gibson, O (2009) *'Government forced to bail out major Olympic projects.'* The Guardian, 21 January 2009

Gibson, O (2010) *'BBC unveils slimmed down World Cup squad of 295 (plus a flatpack studio).'* The Guardian, 12 March 2010

Gibson, O (2012) *'BBC sports chief underlines commitment to the big events.'* The Guardian, 26 April 2012

Gibson, O (2012b) *'BBC Olympic staff to outnumber Team GB athletes.'* The Guardian, 25 April 2012

Gibson, O (2013) *'ESPN apologises after commentator calls Liverpool's Luis Suarez a 'cheat'.'* The Guardian, 7 January 2013

Gibson, O (2014) *'Manchester City ponder FFP appeal after UEFA makes final offer.'* The Guardian, 9 May 2014

Gibson, O (2014b) *'You take sport off free-to-air TV at your peril.'* The Guardian, 5 February 2014

Gibson, O (2015a) *'Sky and BT retain Premier League TV rights for a record £5.14 billion.'* The Guardian, 10 February 2015

Gibson, O (2015b) *'BT executive says Premier League deal vindicate entry into market.'* The Guardian, 11 February 2015

Gibson, O (2015c) *'How IMG spread Premier League's global brand – from a trading estate near Heathrow.'* The Guardian, 01 April 2015

Gibson, O (2015d) *'BBC dealt another blow after losing control of TV rights for Olympics.'* The Guardian, 29 June 2015

Gilpin, R (2001) *Global Political Economy, understanding the international economic order.* Princeton: Princeton University Press

Giulianotti, R (1999) *Football: a sociology of the global game,* Cambridge: Polity

Giulianotti, R (2005) *'Playing an Aerial Game: The New Political Economy of Soccer',* in Nauright, J and K Schimmel (eds) (2005) The Political Economy of Sport. London: Palgrave MacMillan pp 19–37

Glendenning, B (2013) *'BT Sport takes on Sky with a tweak rather than a dramatic upheaval.'* The Guardian, 17 August 2013

Goldlust, J (1987) *Playing for keeps: sport, the media and society.* Melbourne: Longman Cheshire

Goodley, S and A Monaghan (2013) *'BSkyB could face Premier League premium.'* The Guardian, 11 November 2013

Gratton C and H A Solberg (2004) *'Sports and Broadcasting: Comparisons between the United States and Europe',* in International Sports Economics Comparisons, eds R Fort and J Fitzel. Westport, CT and London: Praeger

Gratton, C and H A Solberg (2007) *The Economics of Sports Broadcasting.* London: Routledge

Gruneau, R and H Cantelon (1988) *'Capitalism, commercialism and the Olympics',* in J Seagrave and D Chu (eds), The Olympic Games in transition. Champaign: Human Kinetics, pp 245–64

Harris, N (2012) *'£5.5bn: The staggering sum TV companies around the world will pay to screen the Premier League.'* The Daily Mail, 08 May 2012

Harvey, D (2005) *A Brief History of Neoliberalism*. Oxford; Oxford University Press

Haynes, R (2005) *Media Rights and Intellectual Property*. Edinburgh; Edinburgh University Press

HBS (2013) Available online at www.hbs.tv/host-broadcast-services/about-us/company-profile.html [Accessed 19 December 2013]

Herman, E S and R W McChesney (1997) *The Global Media: the new missionaries of corporate capitalism*. London: Cassell

Hewlett, S (2012) *'Ofcom's tussle with BSkyB leaves it in a terrible position.'* The Guardian, 12 August 2012

Hewlett, S (2013) *'BT may have beaten Sky on Champions League – but the game isn't over.'* The Guardian, 24 November 2013

Holt, R (1989) *Sport and the British, a Modern History*. Oxford: Oxford University Press

Holt, R and T Mason (2000) *Sport in Britain 1945–2000*. Oxford: Blackwell Publishing

Horsman, M (1997) *Sky High*, London: Orion Business Books

Infront (2013) Available online at www.infrontsports.com/production/host-broadcast-services/ [Accessed 3 March 2014]

IOC (2009) Available online at www.olympic.org/uk/organisation/facts/revenue/broadcast_uk [Accessed 1 July 2009]

IOC (2012) Available online at www.olympic.org/sponsors [Accessed 15 October 2012]

Jay, K (2004) *More Than Just a Game. Sports in American Life since 1945*. New York: Columbia University Press

Jeanrenaud, C and S Kesenne (2006) *The Economics of Sport and the Media*, Cheltenham: Edward Elgar

Jenkins, S (2014) *'Winter Olympics: one day the worm will turn against these gods of sport.'* The Guardian, 10 January 2014

Jennings, A (2006) *Foul! The secret world of FIFA: bribes, vote rigging and ticket scandals*. London: HarperCollins

Keter, V and T Jarret (2006) *Transfer of Undertakings (TUPE), Standard Note:SNBT/1064*, London: House of Commons Library

Khalsa, B (2012) *'Endemol closes doors and executives exit.'* Broadcast, 1 February 2012

Magdalinski, T, K S Schimmel and T J L Chandler (2005) *'Recapturing Olympic Mystique: The Corporate Invasion of the Classroom'* in J Nauright and K S Schimmel (eds) (2005) The Political Economy of Sport. Basingstoke: Palgrave MacMillan

Mance, H (2014) *'Ofcom to review Sky's Sports dominance.'* The Financial Times, 16 April 2014

Martin, B (2013) *Difficult Men. From The Sopranos and The Wire to Mad Men and Breaking Bad: Behind the Scenes of a Creative Revolution*. London: Faber and Faber

Mason, R and M Moore (2009) *'Setanta collapse leaves millions of sports fans in the dark.'* The Daily Telegraph, 24 June 2009

Mason, S M (1999) *'What is the Sport product and Who Buys it? The Marketing of Professional Sports Leagues'*. European Journal of Marketing (1999), 33(34). MCB: University Press, pp 402–418

McCarthy, T (2014) *'NBC Secures $7.5bn deal to broadcast Olympics through 3032'.* The Guardian, 7 May 2014

McChesney, R W (1989) '*Media Made Sport: A History of Sports Coverage in the United States*', in L A Wenner (ed) (1989) Media Sport and Society. London: Sage, pp 49–69

McChesney, R W (2008) *The Political Economy of the Media; enduring issues, emerging dilemmas*. New York; Monthly Review Press

McGrew, A (2005) '*The Logics of Globalization*', Global Political Economy, John Ravenhill (ed), 208–234, Oxford: Oxford University Press

Mediatique (2005) *From the Cottage to the City: the evolution of the UK Independent Production Sector.* Independent Report Commissioned by the BBC, September 2005. Available online at www.downloads.bbc.co.uk/aboutthebbc/homework/reports/pdf/independent_production.pdf. [Accessed 13 May 2014]

Midgley, N (2015) '*BT TV's Delia Bushell: "We're not on a trolley dash to take all sports rights".*' The Guardian, 14 June 2015.

Milmo, D (2002) '*Sky's grand prix ratings stay in the pits.*' The Guardian, 19 July 2002

Mosco, V (1996) *The Political Economy of Communication.* London: Sage

Mosey, R (2015) '*Despite losing control of rights to the Olympics, all is not lost for the BBC.*' The Guardian, 29 June 2015

Nally, P (1979) *Intersoccer.* Available online at www.westnally.com/past-projects/intersoccer/4 [Accessed 12 May 2014]

Nauright, J (2005) '*Conclusion: The Political Economy of Sport in the Twenty-first Century*', in Nauright, J and K Schimmel eds (2005) The Political Economy of Sport. London: Palgrave MacMillan, pp 208–214

Nauright, J and K Schimmel (eds) (2005*) The Political Economy of Sport.* London: Palgrave MacMillan

Neale, W (1964) '*The Peculiar Economics of Professional Sports*' Quarterly Journal of Economics, 78, pp 1–4

OBS (2013) Available online at www.obs.tv [Accessed 18 December 2013]

Ofcom (2010) *Pay TV Statement.* Available online at www.stakeholders.ofcom.org.uk/consultations/third_paytv/statement. [Accessed 10 May 2014]

Ofcom (2013) *The Ofcom Broadcasting Code. Available online at* http://stakeholders.ofcom.org.uk/broadcasting/broadcast-codes/broadcast-code/ [Accessed 23 November 2013]

OTAB (2013) Available online at www.otab.com. [Accessed 21 November 2013]

Owen, B and S Wildman (1992) *Video Economics*, Cambridge: Harvard University Press

Peck, T (2015) '*Premier League TV rights: Sky Sports and BT Sport win UK broadcasting rights as price tops £5 billion.*' The Independent, 10 February 2015

Perelman, M (2012) *Barbaric Sport, A Global Plague.* London: Verso

Picard, R (1989) *Media Economics, Concepts and Issues.* London: Sage

PL (2015) Premier League awards UK live broadcast rights for 2016/17 to 2018/19 Available online at www.premierleague.com/en-gb/news/news/2014-15/feb/100215-premier-league-uk-live-broadcasting-rights-announced.html [Accessed 3 July 2015]

Pope, S W (1997) *Patriotic Games. Sporting Traditions in the American Imagination.* New York. Oxford University Press

Press Association (2012) '*Premier League sells domestic TV rights to Sky and BT for £3.018bn*'. The Guardian, 13 June 2012

PwC (2015) *PwC Outlook for the global sports market to 2015*. Available online at http://www.pwc.com/gx/en/hospitality-leisure/changing-the-game-outlook-for-the-global-sports-market-to-2015.jhtml [Accessed 10 July 2015]

Quirk J and R Fort (1992) *Pay Dirt: The Business of Professional Team Sports*. Princeton, New Jersey: Princeton University Press

Quirk J and R Fort (1999) *Hardball: The Abuse of Power in Pro Sports*. Princeton, New Jersey: Princeton University Press

Rankin, J (2013) *'Market for TV sport hit record £16bn in 2014 as broadcasters play hardball.'* The Guardian, 03 January 2014

Robinson, J (2009) *'ESPN wins Premier League football rights.'* The Guardian, 22 June 2009

Rottenberg, S (1956) *'The Baseball Players' Labor Market'*, Journal of Political Economy 64, pp 242–258

Sale, C (2013) *'BT Sport red-faced after SECOND crude gesture on live TV...just 24 hours after Ginola's gaff'*, Mail Online, 22 November 2013. Available online at www.dailymail.co.uk/sport/football/article-2471358/BT-Sport-left-red-faced-second-pundit-makes-crude-gesture-days.html [Accessed 22 October 2013]

Sale, C (2014) *'Richard Scudamore sexism row almost ignored by Rupert Murdoch's empire.'* Daily Mail, 18 May 2014

Sale, C (2014b) *'BT to show ex-ref Halsey the red card after alleged bow to Premier League pressure.'* The Daily Mail, 20 February 2014

Sale, C (2015) *'Sky Sports forced into making cuts after new Premier League TV rights deal.'* The Daily Mail, 01 April 2015

Scannel, P and D Cardiff (1991) *A Social History of British broadcasting: 1922–1939 Serving the Nation Vol 1*, Oxford: Wiley-Blackwell

Schimmel, K (2005) *'Sport and International Political Economy: An Introduction'*, in Nauright, J and K Schimmel (eds) (2005) The Political Economy of Sport. London: Palgrave MacMillan, pp 1–15

Sendall, B (1982) *Independent Television in Britain: Volume 1: Origin and Foundation 1946–62*. London: Macmillan

Sherwin, A (2014) *'Clare Balding and Charles Dance lead BBC's digitally-enabled Sochi 2014 Olympics coverage,'* The Independent, 9 January 2014

Simson, V and A Jennings (1992) *Dishonored Games. Corruption, Money and Greed at the Olympics*. Toronto: Stoddart

Smit, B (2006) *Pitch Invasion, adidas, puma and the making of modern sport*. London: Penguin Books

Smith, P (2009) *The Politics of Sports Rights: The Regulation of Television Sports Rights in the United Kingdom*, paper, Department of Media, Film and Journalism, Faculty of Humanities, De Montfort University

Smythe, D (1977) *'Communications: Blindspot of Western Marxism'* Canadian Journal of Political and Social Theory, 1(3), pp 1–27

Solberg (2006) *'International Television Sports Rights: Risky Investments'* in Jeanrenaud C, and S Kesenne (eds) (2006) The Economics of Sport and the Media. Cheltenham: Edward Elgar, pp 106–125

Solberg, H A and C Gratton (2000) *'The Economics of TV-Sports Rights – The Case of European Soccer'*, European Journal for Sport Management, 7, Special Edition, pp 69–98

Spence, A M and B M Owen (1975, 1977) *'Television Programming, Monopolistic Competition and Welfare'*, Quarterly Journal of Economics 91, pp 103–126

Spence, J (1988) *Up Close & Personal, The Inside Story of Network Television Sports*, New York, New York: Athenium

Stanford, (2010) Available online at www.facultygsb.stanford.edu/mcmillan/personal_page/documents/Bidding%20for%20Olympic%20Broadcast%20Rights.pdf [Accessed 17 August 2010]

Strange, S (1986) *Casino Capitalism*. New York: Basil Blackwell

Sugden J and A Tomlinson (eds) (1998) *FIFA and the Contest for World Football* Cambridge: Polity Press

Sweney, M (2009) *'BSkyB wins Premier League TV rights package back from Setanta.'* The Guardian, 6 February 2009

Sweney, M (2009b) *'Wimbledon's John Rowlinson to be broadcast head for 2012 Olympics.'* The Guardian, 28 April 2009

Sweney, M (2012) *'BT Vision's Marc Watson: How we stole a share of the Premier League crown jewels.'* The Guardian, 1 July 2012

Sweney, M (2013) *'William Morris Endeavour and Silver Lake buy IMG Worldwide for $2.3bn.'* The Guardian, 18 December 2013

Sweney, M (2014) *'All3Media sold to Discovery and Liberty Global in deal worth £500m.'* The Guardian, 8 May 2014

Sweney, M (2014b) *'BSkyB profits hit by cost of Premier League deal.'* The Guardian, 30 January 2014

Sweney, M (2015a) *'Sky adds 127,000 customers in third quarter.'* The Guardian, 21 April 2015

Sweney, M (2015b) *'Channel 5 to show Football League highlights in prime-time Saturday slot.'* The Guardian, 05 May 2015

Szymanski (2006) *'Why Have Premium Sports Rights Migrated to Pay-TV in Europe But Not in the US?* In Jeanrenaud C, and S Kesenne (eds) (2006) The Economics of Sport and the Media. Cheltenham: Edward Elgar, pp 148–159

Todreas, T M (1999) *Value Creation and Branding in Television's Digital Age.* Westport, Connecticut: Quorum Books

Transfer of Undertakings (Protection of Employment) Regulations 2006. Available online at www.legilsation.gov.uk/uksi/2006/246/contents/made [Accessed 12 May 2014]

Tunstall, J (1993) *Television Producers.* London: Routledge

UEFA (2009) Available online at www.uefa.com/uefa/keytopics/kind=131072/index.html [Accessed 7 July 2009]

UEFA (2011) *UEFA Champions League Production Manual.* Available online at http://com23.es/invitado/Master/UCL_Production_Manual_2011%20121.pdf [Accessed 14 October 2013]

UEFA (2013) *Financial Fair Play.* Available online at www.uefa.org/footballfirst/protectingthegame/financialfairplay/ [Accessed 21 October 2013]

Van Wijk, J (2013) *'BT reveal they are considering bid for Champions League football to rival ITV and Sky Sports.'* The Independent, 10 October 2013

Whannel, G (1992) *Fields in Vision. Television sport and cultural transformation.* London: Routledge

Whitson, D (1998) *'Circuits of promotion: media, marketing and the globalization of sport'*, in L A Wenner (ed) (1998), Mediasport. London: Routledge, pp 57–72

Williams, C (2013) *'BT admits failings as BT Sport causes surge in complaints.'* The Telegraph, 13 December 2013

Williams, C (2014) *'Premier League aims to pit BSkyB against BT in early TV rights sale.'* The Telegraph, 8 January 2014

WTO, (2004) Available online at www.wto.org [Accessed 10 July 2012]

Zeigler, M (2013) *'New Premier League TV deal promises £100m prize money for next season's title winners,* The Telegraph, 21 May 2013

Index

Printed in the United States
By Bookmasters